Fat to Fab

By
Tobi Beck, PhD, JD

Beckenhall Publishing
Distribution by Lulu.com

Beckenhall Publishing, Avon, IN
First Edition 2010 – Electronic
Second Edition 2012 – Electronic and Paperback

ISBN 978-0- 09669399-3-X

Dedication

First, this is dedicated to my Husband, who is encouraging, loving and wonderful in every way,

Second, to my proofreaders Steve and Kathy and Nancy,

And most importantly: To the Amazing Shrinking Friends, who did me the honor of allowing me to change their lives.

Table of Contents

It's Time to Try Something Else

I'm torn. How do I get across to you all of the incredible things that this program does, without sounding too good to be true? If you believe that what I say is hype, you will put this down and never look at it again, and miss the opportunity to change your life, and I will have done you a disservice. If I fail to tell you all that the program can do, I've done you a different disservice. Do I highlight that the program is a fix for the root cause of weight gain, and when it is fixed, like any bone or organ or other damage to the body, you return to a normal life? Do I point out that your body is fixing itself the way it was designed to do, and, also as it was designed to do, the body will retract the skin along with dissolving the fat? Do I highlight that because we are not attempting to change the metabolism (your body will do that by itself) there is no strenuous exercise in this program - no metabolism boosters? Because you are not depriving your body of what it needs there are no fat blockers,   no starch blockers, no pills? Would you laugh and declare it is impossible if I explained that you won't be hungry while doing the program, because your body is being fed from the fat stores? Do I dare to point out that it works for every person, every time? Would you believe that there may be a CURE for obesity? Can you believe each of those statements? Can you dare to hope, again, that it is possible?

Dr. Simeons, the author of the original protocol titled "Pounds and Inches – a new approach to obesity" writes that his struggle to find and cure the disease 'obesity' was "a long series of high hopes and bitter disappointments." The same can be true for all of us who have attempted to lose weight.

This program is based on Dr. Simeons' work, and updated with the experiences of The Shrinking Friends team who put the protocol to the test, in a modern world. In many cases, I've referenced Dr. Simeons' words directly, where he is readily understandable, such as when he discusses this program as a cure, and why he classified this as a cure;

"If this reasoning is correct, it follows that a treatment aimed at curing the disorder must be equally effective in both sexes, at all ages and in all forms of obesity. Unless this is so, we are entitled to harbor grave doubts as to whether a given treatment corrects the underlying disorder. Moreover, any claim that the disorder has been corrected must be substantiated by the ability of the patient to eat normally of any food he pleases without regaining Abnormal fat after treatment. Only if these conditions are fulfilled can we legitimately speak of curing obesity rather than of reducing weight."

Where he is less obvious in what he writes, I've simply provided an interpretation for the layman such as:

"That this is the true mechanism underlying the presumed gonadotrophic action of HCG is confirmed by the fact that when the pituitary gland of infantile rats is removed before they are given HCG, the latter has no effect on their sex-glands. HCG cannot therefore have a direct sex gland stimulating action like that of the anterior pituitary gonadotrophins, as FSH and LSH are justly called. The latter are entirely different substances from that which can be extracted from pregnancy urine and which, unfortunately, is called chorionic gonadotrophin. It would be no more clumsy, and certainly far more appropriate, if HCG were henceforth called chorionic dienccphalotrophin."

Which is to say: HCG is kind of misnamed in the health community and therefore often mistaken as a hormone exclusively linked to pregnancy and sexual development.

It actually works the same in both men and women, old and young. A detailed explanation of why can be found in the protocol. The original protocol is printed in its entirety in the back of the book. Some of the medical beliefs of fifty years ago, such as the origin of HCG, have changed. However, the effectiveness of the program has not.

You may be skeptical, like the vast majority who have tried other weight loss plans, diets, exercise, equipment, metabolism boosters, fat blockers, food programs, hypnosis, you name it……there are plenty out there. The problem with all of them is that they do not fix the problem. Some will tell you they will fix the problem by fixing your metabolism, but unless you correct the part of the body that regulates the metabolism, that diet – like any other that fights the body – will eventually fail. This program is aimed at fixing the body regulator. Once healed, you will have the weight you want, the body you never thought you would see, and be able to eat as you wish, and keep both. Yes, it sounds too good to be true. It is good, and it is true.

If I told you there was a weight loss program out there that:
- involved little exercise, and even that was optional,
- provided rapid weight loss, about a pound a day,
- was inexpensive,
- required little willpower,
- involved no hunger,
- helped you to feel great doing it, and look healthy and vibrant throughout,
- allowed you to select your weight,
- shrank the skin, along with the weight,
- kept the weight off when you finished, while eating what you want, and
- worked for every person, every time, no matter how overweight you were,

You would tell me it was too good to be true. And I would have agreed, until I lost over 60 pounds in less than 6 months and felt great doing it. I wanted to make sure it wasn't just me, so I shared with my friends, and fewer than 50 people lost over a ton of weight. Literally a ton - over 2,000 pounds in less than six months.

I was sure the weight would all come back. It did not. I was sure it was too good to be true. It wasn't. I was sure it would not work for everyone. It did. Up until now this program was available at an expensive weight loss clinic in Europe (Salvator Mundi International Hospital in Rome). It's been available for more than half a century there. This is the first step by step guide to doing this program at home, for yourself. This book will take you through how to reset your body weight for life, no matter how much you have to lose, no matter how old you are, no matter if you don't believe. Every other program out there is about fighting your body by temporarily increasing your metabolism, blocking starches or fats or burning more calories and taking in less food. This program is about resetting your body, working with it, not against it, and returning you to a life without weight watching.

We all complain about the epidemic of obesity. Most of us are overweight, but nothing we have tried has worked to take it off. Maybe that's because we are trying the wrong thing. Maybe it is because what we have been taught (reduce calories, diet and exercise, increase metabolism, block starches, replace sugar….etc.) is wrong. Maybe it is time to fix the problem, the weight regulator in the body itself, rather than treat the symptoms of being overweight. This book will show you how.

Everything you need is in these pages. If you have the book and want additional help, it is available. If you want a group and personal guide, who has already done this program, to answer questions and walk you through the program, we have that. Some people work better this way, and it is about getting you to the weight you want, the best way that works for you. You can drop me a note at Tobi@fat2fab.org and I'll work with you to join the Facebook page of the Amazing Shrinking Friends. It is a great place to ask questions, find reassurance and share with others, and generally provides a go-to place for any concerns. Consider checking out the site, or even signing up for a team, they are there for you.

This program is about choice. You get to choose what weight you want to be in the end, as long as it is still in the healthy range – the program will not let you lose healthy fat. You can choose how much detail you want to know about the program, you can choose to cheat, you can even choose to skip ahead and review only the parts that interest you. However, when presented with such choices, you should know there are consequences; so wherever possible, we have tried to outline the consequences so that you can make an informed choice. Here is your first one: you can choose to skip ahead and read only the parts that interest you. I will tell you that the most successful people read the whole plan, including the original protocol and commit to it before starting. It is an easy read and a little dedication in this area will set you up for success. However, if you must, here is a quick list of the most likely places of interest.

If you want just the program step by step start on page 56.
If you want just the food list go to page 63.
If you want to know why it works start on page 22.
If you want to see how it worked for others go to page 93.
If you want to know why other diets don't work that's on page 27.
If you want recipes they start on page 120.
If you want the original Dr.'s Protocol it starts on page 168.

This is not a book about how the suspect marketing practices of fast food chains make it easy to overeat, or the additives they put in the food to addict the average person. This is not about how the weight loss industry as a whole keeps us in a cycle of Loss -> Gain -> Gain Additional Weight -> New program -> Loss...... This is not about the latest fad in exercise equipment to 'reduce those love handles' or pills to 'rev up your metabolism.' While all those products are out there, and the various industries do some amazing things to make a profit, that is not the main topic of this book. This book is about how to adjust your body's weight regulator, and have your body heal itself. The premise starts with the idea that the system that regulates your weight is damaged; otherwise you would not be overweight. Fix the organ/system, and fix the weight. Fail to fix the organ/system and nothing you do will be a permanent solution for your weight issues.

The definition of insanity is trying the same thing and expecting a different result. If the diets of the past have failed......perhaps we need to change what we think we know about weight loss. As a rule we are told that a reduced-calorie diet of healthy food and vigorous exercise will reduce our weight and give us the ideal model body. The problem is, permanent weight loss is achieved by less than one tenth of one percent of people using this guideline. It's heart-wrenching for me to see significantly overweight people out jogging, doing their best to follow the conventional wisdom of diet and exercise. They try so hard, they are clearly in pain, they suffer significantly, and the results are minor. They become disappointed, and stop soon enough. They regain any weight they lost and then a little more. All the while, I know that just a portion of that dedication could have yielded significant weight loss results, had they followed the program outlined here.

We are also repeatedly told that no sudden loss of weight can be permanent. In a conventional diet, this would be true. However, the conventional diet attempts to fool the body into a temporary reaction, whereas this program is about permanent change.

The thinking behind the program is unconventional, but we already know that conventional does not work. The first thing to come to terms with is the idea that being overweight is not your fault. Conventional wisdom tells us that those who overeat are overweight, that it is a result of being lazy or indulging in excess. We have only recently learned that this is not the case at all. We live in a world where the very food we eat has additives and chemicals that cause us to gain weight. Recent studies sponsored by the government have shown a new class of chemical in our food called 'obesogens' that increase our natural ability to gain weight. [1] Dr. Simeons theorized that being overweight was caused by an imbalance in the endocrine system and the hypothalamus, which regulates it. The hypothalamus is an almond-sized portion in the middle of the brain that controls metabolism, body temperature, thirst, hunger and other autonomic functions; it is also the body's weight regulator. This imbalance may be due to the chemicals in the highly processed and preserved food that is readily available today at the supermarket and fast food chains.

Through exhaustive research, which he outlines in the protocol, Dr. Simeons theorized that as an act of self-preservation the human body provides a fully-functioning endocrine system as an early priority during pregnancy. He also discovered that a small amount of HCG (about 1/1000 of what a pregnant woman produces daily) will cause the body to repair and reset the hypothalamus and endocrine system. This works in both men and women, without feminizing men or maculating women.

In the 1950's Dr. Simeons moved his research in obesity into practice, opening a clinic in Europe. He ultimately wrote Pounds & Inches, A new Approach to Obesity as a guide for other doctors opening clinics to treat patients as he had done for the previous 15 years. In recent years, through the advent of the Internet, the transcript has become

---

[1]   White House Study released May 11, 2010 "Solving the Problem of Childhood Obesity within a Generation".

widely available. It is, however written by a doctor, for other doctors, as an instruction in how to conduct a clinic. The directions for mixing and dosing can be confusing, and the idea of self-administered injections is a little scary. Further, there are a few things addressed only obliquely in the original protocol that we will bring out in detail here.

Here for the first time is an interpretation for the layman. For you, as a guide to treat yourself to the benefits of a world-renowned obesity treatment center, without staying at a private hospital or traveling to Europe. The process is detailed, though not difficult to follow. There are directions for mixing the injections as in the original protocol, and dosing for drops administered under the tongue. The supplement is easy to obtain and inexpensive. The food is readily available at your local supermarket. And people just like you share their insights, tips and experiences. In short, everything you need to take off the fat and keep it off for life is at hand. The plan is inexpensive, and with this book as a guide, you can do this at home. This book goes well beyond Dr. Simeons' protocol in that it gives you, the average person, the knowledge and ability to take this on yourself, without a clinic. Also included are testimonials, before and after pictures, recipes and other tidbits of information that you will find, if not inspirational, certainly useful.

There are no long-term counseling programs and dues to pay for, no prepackaged food programs to subscribe to, and no exercise program or gym memberships or special equipment to 'target trouble areas.' The program takes the excess weight off, takes it from all the problem areas, won't let you lose healthy weight, retracts the skin where the weight came off, drops weight quickly and resets the body to maintain a new weight. There are no expensive commitments or equipment, or even a strenuous exercise program. The program has a beginning and a definite end, after which you return to a normal eating routine, and life. Let me be clear...no supplements to take for life, no diets to maintain, no exercise programs to be slave to...none. The body has amazing resilience and can be healed. This program is about healing the body. Not through vigorous exercise or metabolism boosters but through a program that fixes the system that regulates the body. When you are down to a healthy weight, then pick up an exercise program and go after a well muscled beach body, if that's what you choose; but for now, let's take the first things first., Let's get the weight off.

There are all sorts of conspiracy theories as to why this has not become available to the public before. Some say the diet food industry did its best to keep it out of the public's hands, because it would forever eliminate the need to be on another diet. Certainly there is no one to champion this work, as there is no money to be made from a simple, inexpensive long term solution when it is more lucrative to sell something less effective and more expensive. Once the program is followed, the person is finished. The weight does not come back, and if it starts to the person can easily   conduct another round to return to their new, desired weight quickly and simply. It is not surprising, then, that some have suggested that the diet food industry actively tries to block this information. Who would blame them if they did? After all, it would put them out of business. But I don't think it is that sinister. It is more likely that the plan is just not widely known, and it goes against conventional wisdom, so it is not widely promoted. It does not take a rocket scientist to figure out that conventional wisdom as it stands is not curing people of being overweight. The problem is in epidemic proportions, and all the standard answers are not working to solve the problem. So maybe we need to go back to the root cause of the problem, and fix that.

While the program was designed and tested initially by a doctor, he is not your doctor. While this program can be done at home, you should consult your doctor, have them read the original protocol and take into consideration your particular circumstances. To date we have not had a single doctor who read the protocol suggest that losing weight with this program would be worse than keeping the weight. Several doctors joined us after seeing the results in their patients. Consult your doctor, particularly if you take blood pressure medication, heart medication, diabetes medication or any other medication that is prescribed based on your weight. On this program your weight drops quickly and your weight-based medication must be monitored, and may need to be adjusted (or eliminated) to compensate. Several members on the team drastically reduced heart, diabetes, thyroid and pain medication while following the plan protocol. Several doctors indicated that while they could not recommend the program because of restrictions of the institution that they worked for, they did not dissuade those who asked about it. Those in private practice simply agreed that it was worth a try. If you have any concerns, consult with your doctor.

That said, I'm glad you can join us. My goal is to have everyone at the weight they choose to be.

Welcome aboard!

Dieting Should Not Be This Hard

Growing up I wasn't one of the popular people in high school. I was always a little overweight, big in the hips and thighs, not really fat, but not the ideal of beauty either. I joined the military and exercised regularly and even at my healthiest, I struggled to keep my weight within acceptable range for the rigid standards. When I left the military I slowly gained weight, about a half pound a month or so, nothing dramatic, but it was steady.

I dieted, exercised, tried one program after another, but it always came back. After a while, I started to see doctors with the specific intent of finding a reason for my constant weight gain. It wasn't much, but it was constant, and I couldn't make it stop. Half a pound a month does not seem like much, but that is 60 pounds in 10 years. I couldn't simply accept gaining weight as a side effect of getting older. I had a ghost breathing over my shoulder – my mother died weighing over 650 pounds. When I expressed my concern to the doctor, he told me not to worry. Too late.

I went to clinics and nutritionists and was told to keep a diary of what food I ate and what exercise I did. After a while I would just hand them the previous six month's records on the spot when asked to keep such a diary. Invariably they would review it and tell me that I was cheating on what I was recording. I wasn't. And then I would go to the next one.

I tried food programs, specific food diets, exercise programs and clinic gimmicks, including one that determined how many calories you should eat based on how much oxygen you processed with each breath. I always felt deprived, and they were never successful for very long. I even considered plastic surgery. I ate moderately and healthily and exercised regularly, and I still could not stop the relentless gain.

When I went to the last doctor I saw while attempting to find a way to lose weight, I told him about all my efforts, and found myself just short of tears as I confessed how many ways I had failed. He was a reasonably fit man, something I noticed was harder and harder to find among doctors these days, and I hardly expected him to believe me. I was even a little embarrassed and surprised at my own emotional reaction. He looked me in the eye, smiled warmly and simply said: "Losing weight shouldn't be this hard, should it?" I was shocked! He heard me, and he actually appreciated what I was feeling. That's fairly rare in a doctor in these times of "treat them and send them home;" actually listening to the patient, and understanding, not just sympathizing or placating, or worse yet, dismissing. He wrote the prescription for HCG, told me where to read the whole protocol and assured me that if I followed it exactly, I would probably never need to talk to him again. I asked how he was so sure. He smiled slowly, knowingly, and pulled a picture out of his wallet. It was him, about a hundred pounds heavier.

I'm a fairly educated person, and while none of my degrees are in medicine I have an understanding of the medical community and the vocabulary used, I understood the protocol. I began the program in early December, and was surprised that no one said anything. In fact, I dropped close to 15 pounds before one of my co-workers, who I had commiserated with about relentless weight gain at one point, realized that I had lost weight, and wanted to know how. I walked her through it, helped her work out the details and start the program herself. Her every victory was mine as well and I began to share with everyone who would listen.

Most thought it was too good to be true, but they could not deny the results. Most of us at work had complained about our weight at one point or another, but we just couldn't change it. One by one I coached more friends through the program, and they began to lose weight quickly. We could see the results on each other. I went from 215 pounds to 152 pounds. I was a size 16+ and went to a size 4 jean.

But I wasn't the only one; B went from 215 to 181 in her first six weeks, Kathy H. dropped 23 pounds her first round, Kim shed an excess 22 pounds. It worked for all age groups; Crystal is in her twenties and lost 25 pounds, Nancy is in her fifties and lost over 50 pounds, Kathy H.T. is in her sixties and lost 60 pounds. It worked for men (actually better); Reed went from 245 to 195, Tim lost 34 pounds his first 6 weeks, Savaric lost 49 pounds. People who were taking medications found they took less or needed to stop. Angie had been on heart and blood pressure medication for 12 years. After the first round she lost 32 pounds, and her doctor took her off all of her medication. Nancy F. had been on the maximum dose of morphine and other pain-management medication for years. Halfway through her first round she realized she needed less, and by the time her first round was through she was down to a third of what she had been taking. Again, she made adjustments under her doctor's supervision.

Seeing is believing. That, if for no other reason, is why there are pictures of 'before' and 'after,' including mine. These are not touched up photos, or ones where you are looking at two different people...they are people like you and me. You will see them shrink, get better posture, and change their shape. Believe one more time. Try one more time...it will be the last time you need to.

Why This Book Is Different

Why is this book different? Because the book is not about dieting. This book is about fixing the root cause of what caused you to be overweight to begin with...and it's not what we have been told. It's also not written by someone talking about theory, averages or research. It is written by someone who did it. According to those horrid height/weight charts, I was obese. Today, according to the same chart, I'm at a healthy weight. I coached others through the process and found that it worked every time, for every person. The book has the words of people who did this, their pictures, their tips, their doubts and their discoveries. The program works, every time when it is followed.

In these pages you will find not just the program to change your weight, but how others like you progressed and moved quickly from fat to fabulous and stayed that way. Yes, you read that right...stayed that way. This is not a diet. If it were, you would feel deprived, low on energy and put the weight back on a few weeks later.

This is a fix for the damaged organ and system that controls your weight. Your body knows what weight it should be, and it returns there at every chance. When we force it below that line for any length of time the body struggles to maintain, and eventually wins out, and packs on a few extra pounds to prevent that kind of scare again. This is about adjusting the weight back to that which your body wants to be. It is done in six week increments, each one resetting the body weight lower. In between loss cycles the new body weight is maintained without great effort, or restriction of food. This is due to the body having a new set weight, one that it wants to return to.

In addition, and as important as the weight loss, is the change in shape. For a number of reasons, a person can be out of proportion. This program redistributes healthy fat and provides a more ideal finished shape. Among the Shrinking Friends, we found this to be exactly true. On days there was not loss in weight, there was a significant change in measurements at the end of the week.

It's hard to believe, particularly if you have tried one or a dozen diets in the past and still can't lose weight and keep it off. Because we have tried the hard diets and they didn't work. It is counterintuitive that something that is easy and quick would have the result we have been searching for. The very thought of being able to eat what you want and not gain weight is unbelievable. But you have seen it. We all know someone who does not exercise much, eats constantly and never seems to gain a pound. This is a person who already healed that organ, or never had it damaged to begin with. You're about to become one of those people. Not overnight, but faster than you ever thought possible.

This book will also cover misconceptions about weight and weight loss, the lies we have come to believe to help us accept our obesity, and why we often don't want to lose weight. We will cover why diets in the past have not worked. You can already guess part of it – they did not address the root cause, but there is more than that to address. The reactions you will receive will be stunning, and we will cover what those around you are likely to say – not all the reactions will be positive, and knowing how to answer them will be key to staying on track. The book includes a step-by-step process of how to work through the diet, recipes to make sure the food stays interesting, and where to go for help should you have any questions, problems or concerns as you progress. This should not be considered a substitute for a doctor's advice. If you have any doubt, worry or concern about your particular health, medication or problems, see your doctor. Those doctors who take the time to read and understand the protocol are almost invariably behind it.

Root Cause

Mostly we live in a world where we fix the symptom, but only once it causes enough discomfort that people seek help. I have heartburn, so I take an antacid. I have a headache, so I take an aspirin. I have dry skin, so I use a lotion. We don't, however, usually look any further for a root cause. What caused the heartburn, headache or dry skin? All too often we are taught to relieve the symptom, and accept that it is simply a sign of getting old, or a normal, if inconvenient, fact of life, or we have a 'condition' and we just have to live with it. We are told that it happens to everyone, and as proof, we have a wide variety of remedies available over–the-counter, and everyone we know has experienced it. But, again, we don't look further for the root cause. When the symptom is more serious, we seek immediate attention and treat the symptom, because to do otherwise would be life threatening. High blood pressure? Diabetes? Heart problems? We take medication to bring us back to normal, but we don't fix the problem that caused it……the diabetic patient knows they need to lose weight but the Doctor usually prescribes diet and exercise or some other program that would treat the symptom of obesity, but not the cause.

This habit is particularly devastating when it comes to weight. Some say they are fixing the root cause by increasing the metabolism "so that your body turns into a fat-burning machine." The problem is that if you don't correct the metabolism regulator, anything you do to temporarily adjust your metabolism will eventually be overcome by your amazingly resourceful body. As a result, whatever you have done to adjust yourself will eventually stop working. When it does, the weight regulator in the body (the hypothalamus) returns us to our unnatural 'set' weight. Then, to add indignity, the body packs on a few more pounds to protect itself from any future sudden loss like that.

Many studies show that most people are overweight, and it is a growing problem. It's all around us and has become acceptable. In a single night of TV you can see a dozen commercials for weight loss products. There are fat blockers, starch blockers, diet teas, metabolism boosters, eating programs, counseling programs, prepackaged foods, diet fads and even exercise programs used to 'trim down those unwanted love handles.' But not one of them actually addresses the root cause of the problem. We are told that being overweight is a result of overeating or lack of exercise. Or as recent government studies have suggested, there are hidden 'obesigens' in our food sources[2]. Others suggest that the epidemic in obesity came about with the introduction of the food pyramid, which strongly encouraged the consumptions of grains and gluten[3]. Most people still have a belief that being overweight is a result of overeating and they look with disgust at every mouthful they see an obese person eat.

 Dr. Simeons, on the other hand, theorized that overeating was a result of being overweight, instead of being the cause. The obese person ate more, because they needed more fuel to perform the same functions that a thin person can do with less fuel. The obese person's bodies have more mass to cool and heat and move, all of which takes more fuel.

What is the cause? Dr. Simeons theorized that, *in every case*, the cause of being overweight is a result of a damaged hypothalamus. The greater the damage, the faster a person gains weight, and the

---

[2] Ibid.

[3] David S. Ludwig, Children's Hospital Boston, Journal of the American Medical Association, May 2002.

more overweight they are and stay.   Because being overweight is a result of a damaged organ, the solution works the same on all people, male and female, no matter how great the obesity.   Fix the hypothalamus, fix the obesity.   Once fixed, the person can return to eating what they wish and not regain the weight.

Dr. Simeons set out to perfect the program, and did. While it was created many years ago (in the early '50s), the program works and has worked for hundreds of thousands of people. It worked for me, and I shared it with my friends. I coached them through the program, exactly as this book is coaching you now, and it does work, every time, for every person, when they followed the program. Better than just taking weight off easily, the weight stays off, because the root cause is fixed. This book updates what Dr. Simeons discovered, modernizes many of his observations backed by additional case studies, translates how to apply the program at home instead of in a European clinic and provides the whole study in layman's terms. The book is, in short, all you will need to succeed on this program.

The program is not difficult. It is, however, precise. No variation is acceptable, *no matter how well justified or intellectually rationalized*. It works, it is not expensive, it will take the weight off quickly and keep it off for life. Each detail is outlined here, and as you progress through the program you will find that it works exactly as specified.   Doing this program at home requires that you believe and follow the details exactly. There will be points where a detail seems trivial, or excessive; it is not. It is up to you to follow the rules.

Why Diets Fail

Remember, this is not a diet. It is a recovery plan for the hypothalamus. The good news is that as we fix the hypothalamus, your weight also corrects itself, and like healing any part of the body, the results are quick. The original protocol explains in great detail the bodily processes, and if you want more detail, please read Dr. Simeons' protocol. What follows is a more simplified, though complete, synopsis.

In order to explain why diets fail, we have to look at how the body sees fat. There are three types of fat that the body distinguishes. Structural fat protects the organs, fills out the skin and provides a cushion on the fingertips and bottoms of the feet. Structural fat is necessary for good health. The second type is Normal fat. This is the fat that takes you from day to day and meal to meal with a normal reserve. We contribute and take freely from this reserve to fuel the body on a daily basis. Structural and normal fat together is what should be in the body, and makes up 18-24% in a female and 14-18% in men.

There is however, a third type of fat...Abnormal fat. Think of this as fat locked in the warehouse and stored for a rainy day. Unfortunately, the body is storing it for only the greatest of emergencies and when it does not have any emergencies at hand, the body "forgets" where it stored the fat. First, Abnormal fat is a layer placed all over the body, and secondly this fat is packed on to the areas where we usually want to get rid of it most. For most women this is in the hips, thighs and stomach; for men, it is usually the stomach. The body is most unwilling to give up this last reserve, even when it is the largest available.

How did the Abnormal fat get there to begin with? There are many different ways - stress, a damaged hypothalamus that fails to regulate hunger properly, eating for comfort rather than need and even chemicals in modern food can all contribute.

A diet works on the theory that reducing the calories and increasing the body's demand for the calories will cause the body to dissolve fat to make up the difference. And it does. Unfortunately, the body first dissolves Normal fat, which is the purpose for which this fat was created. Then, when that is exhausted, the body sends out a signal that the fat stores need to be replenished. But this is a diet we are on here, so we ignore those signals and continue to starve the body, at which time the body starts dissolving the Structural fat. In the meantime, the body is busy taking a little from the very inside of the storehouse of Abnormal fat, expecting to return it at the first available opportunity ...with interest. It can do this no faster than a pound or so a week at best. This is why 'healthy' diet programs recommend taking no more than a pound a week. The problem is that the body is only temporarily robbing the storehouse with the intent to replace it at the first opportunity. As soon as any little slip of the diet occurs, the body replaces the storehouse fat first. At the same time the body becomes very efficient at burning calories; after all, it is starving. Like a household with a budget, it has to cut back someplace in order to make ends meet.

As a result, the same diet and exercise routine has reduced effect over time, and in order to maintain or increase a steady loss of weight, the calories need to be reduced, and the exercised continued or increased. The dieter becomes exhausted and hungry because the Normal fat stores are used up and the body wants them replenished. It takes increasing willpower to maintain the diet. Sometimes pain associated to Structural fat loss, such as sore feet, also occurs. One of the Shrinking Friends always had sore feet, and she also dieted constantly, though it did little good. She attributed her near inability to walk to several issues with her feet. Within a few weeks on the program, her feet no longer hurt, and it was more than what losing the weight could have done. The phenomenon was described by Dr. Simeons in section XX. Some few people are able to persevere past this pain and do lose weight this way. They have demonstrated huge feats of will in doing so. Unfortunately, for most of us the body corrects the imbalance in fat stores quickly, and because the storehouse is restored first, the only fat we want to get rid of is the first to come back. In an effort to protect itself from such a starvation in the future, the body adds a few more pounds just to be sure it is protected next time.

People on such diets often look 'hollowed out' or slack-skinned, they are hungry all the time and often irritable. When they do lose enough weight to take from the storehouse, the skin is saggy because the body robbed the storehouse from the inside. For women, one of the first places the body takes from is the Structural fat in the chest, resulting in a very disappointing loss there. Very heavy people lose Structural fat from the bottom of the feet and walking becomes painful; don't even talk about women wearing high heels! After all the dieting, fat still hangs around the places we most want to get rid of it: hips, stomach, and thighs. We've all been here, but you don't have to do that ever again.

How You Will Know This is Not a Diet, But a Recovery

This program will be different, and you will know it quickly. First, unlike a diet, the body will not be taking from normal or Structural fat. In fact, with the HCG the body goes straight after the storehouse fat in an orderly fashion, from the outside in. During the course of the program, the body is consuming 2,500 to 3,000 calories a day, although only 500 of it is coming in between the teeth. The rest is coming from the previously inaccessible storehouse of Abnormal fat.

You will know it is not a diet because your body will not behave like it is a diet.

Because your body will take from the storehouse of Abnormal fat rather than normal or Structural fat, the usual symptoms of being low on normal and Structural fat will not occur. Dr. Simeons points out these features of the program, and the Shrinking Friends team experienced these effects also:

- There won't be hunger, because the body is getting fed 2,500-3,000 calories of fuel a day. In fact, many people on the team just did not want to eat at all.
- The fat will come out of the storehouse, which means off of the waist, hips, thighs and stomach as well as the all-around layer that covers the body. Not the chest for women; in fact, the first place most women show loss is under the chin. Dr. Simeons noted that there was always a regular and dramatic loss in abdominal fat on this program.
- The skin will not get slack, because you are losing it the way your body was made to take it off, from the outside in, retracting the skin as you go.
- The face will not hollow out. That is a result of a starvation diet, a very unhealthy practice, and this is anything but.
- The weight will come off fast, because the body is taking it from the unlocked storehouse at full speed, without attempting to reduce efficiency.

- You will have a great deal of energy rather than lethargy. Because the body is getting plenty of fuel there is plenty of energy.
- Most importantly, the weight will not come back, because the body will reset the weight it wants to return to. This is because the body weight regulator (hypothalamus) has a new and corrected "set" point.

Diets are temporary. This is not. This program fixes the root cause of the problem, and returns you the body you gave up ever having.

We Accept the Weight We Think We Can't Change

Have you heard these?

"I'm naturally a Pear (or Apple) shape."

"Our metabolism slows down after about 30."

"You're just big boned."

"It's hereditary."

"All the women in our family are large."

"Those height/weight charts are old/for insurance agencies/not realistic."

"My metabolism is just slow."

I know I've said most if not all of these things myself. I've been told them by others and we have told these things to each other in an effort to allow us to cope with what we have been unable to change. It is only natural to soothe our egos by giving ourselves a means of accepting the weight. We have a diet industry out there that has a vested interest in making sure that we accept being overweight, and when we want to do something about it, making sure that we try one of their products to take off the weight. The product, food program, counseling program, latest restrictive plan, whatever, will take some off, and put it all back on, as we have discussed already.

We feel that we have failed, because all the commercials show happy successful people (who were probably never on the diet to begin with). We move from one failed diet to another, gaining weight as we go, and lowering self esteem. It seems we have been all but enslaved by a diet industry that binds us to a perpetual cycle.

Is it any wonder that we don't dare try again?

"Diet and Exercise Will Do What I Need."

I used to be a huge fan of diet and exercise. I am ex-Army; of course I believed in diet and exercise - they have you live that reality while on duty. I even went out of my way to learn how to train others, and become an expert in nutrition. I ate healthy food in moderation and exercised on a regular basis. For a while I was even eating a mail order pre-packaged meal plan (about 1,200 calories a day) and exercising up to four hours a day in the gym. My average day was:

> 5:30 Up and bike to the gym.
>
> 6:00 Body Pump ™ workout (fantastic fun by the way).
>
> 7:00 Bike back to apartment, breakfast on plan.
>
> 11:30 Back to the gym for a one hour Spinning ™ class.
>
> 13:00 Quick lunch at the desk (from the plan).
>
> 18:00 Back to gym for yoga or weights.
>
> 20:00 Dinner on plan.
>
> 21:00 Sometimes desert.

After 6 months, I did indeed lose weight, and looked great, and felt fit, if a little tired. But a heavy exercise program and 1,200 calories a day will make you tired. I was a solid gal, and I wasn't at all upset with how I looked. I was still a little disproportionate in the hips and legs, but I was sure that was simply genetic, and I would always be that way. I scoffed at those height/weight charts, because I was in good shape, even though those pesky charts had me as near obese. I was 68" and 180 pounds. In fact, I just could not break that 180 mark, no matter what I did. Unable to get below that 180 mark (the chart says 68" should be between 126 – 167, with a target weight of 146...yeah, right, not in a million years), I tried all sorts of things to help break that plateau. With the above workout and eating program I tried supplements, fat burners, massage, and body wraps, and I'm sure a few other things as well.

I knew there was no lack of will power, no failure to work out, no cheating on the diet...but I didn't drop below 180, so I assumed that the height/weight charts must be totally unreasonable. After all, I'd never been within the chart range for 'healthy' my entire adult life, and I had always considered myself reasonably healthy. Obviously, the chart was wrong (see previous list of lies we tell ourselves). Constant diet and exercise and healthy eating can help a person lose weight, and doing so at the prescribed rate of a pound a week is great. For those who can keep that kind of focus, fantastic. There are a few problems with this approach for most people, though:

1. Most people reach a maximum loss and even if they continue, they just don't lose any more. For me it was still well above what was considered healthy.

2. In addition, it is slow, very slow, and it's difficult to keep motivated....particularly since, depending on the week of the month, you may actually gain a few pounds of water weight, so the scale may not show any progress at all. If you have a hundred pounds to loose, losing at this rate is a multiyear plan. That's a lot of willpower.

3. The whole program all too easily becomes discouraging and the dieter stops; just giving up because there is too much work with not enough result.

4. The new lifestyle has to be maintained, depriving the dieter of time or satisfying food.

5. When the 'diet' is over the weight all comes back on, and it brings a few friends.

What seems to be happening is that the hypothalamus "knows" what weight we should be, and it does everything to keep us there. And, in an overweight person, this "known" weight point has been incorrectly reset. So, when we diet, lose some weight, and then stop the highly restrictive or very active routine, it comes back. Because the hypothalamus recognizes that it could not maintain the 'correct' weight, it puts on a few more pounds, just to make sure it does not go below again....and this becomes the new 'set' weight for the person.

As an overweight person, exercise hurts. The same motion that builds muscle on the fit person is exhausting and in some cases damaging to the extremely heavy. If you are 80 pounds overweight, it is like carrying an 80 pound pack everywhere you go. To give you an idea of the muscles that takes, the average Infantry soldier carries an 80 pound pack for half a day, and is exhausted. The overweight person has to have the same muscle just to move around during the day as that soldier, except they never get to put the pack down. It's not muscle they need to build; it's the proportion of muscle to fat that they need to change. Once the weight is off, exercise will build muscle, and feel great. Until then, it is more physically uncomfortable than it needs to be.

I, like most, was extremely skeptical that the diet could take me below the 180 mark. After all, I had already come to the conclusion that this was the best that I would get, and those charts were just lies. Rest assured, my skepticism was unfounded and I blew past the 180 mark and kept going. In fact, I ended up at the target weight in those pesky weight charts without significant effort or great feats of willpower.

"I Have a Diet Plan That Works Fine For Me."

Fantastic!!!!!! Really, I mean it. If you are losing weight, and you are satisfied with your progress and are able to keep it off after you're finished...great! I'll never tell people that what they are doing is wrong if it is working for them. The end result is a healthier you...and that is what it is all about!

If, on the other hand, the weight comes back, the program is too difficult to maintain for life, you stall in the weight loss, it feels too depriving, or just stops being worth the effort, consider this program. The benefits are many! The program has a finite treatment timeline.

The weight loss is very fast, providing quick progress and motivation. The weight stays off after completing the program and successfully resetting the correct weight. And, after the program, you get to eat what you want, when you want and you don't have to worry about putting the weight back on, because your body has a new 'set' weight that it will naturally want to return to.

There Are Some Unconventional Rules:

Don't Count Calories

I know that this concept is contrary to every diet you've ever tried, or even conventional wisdom, but don't count calories. Calories are important when artificially regulating the body. This program is about having your body regulate itself, naturally, at the weight you want to be. The ability to even judge how many calories are in a particular food is only a recent invention. For this program, just don't do it. Having just said that, there is an exception. The original protocol involved the clinic providing specific portions of foods for the patients, in this way it limited how much of a particular vegetable or fruit was consumed, and the clinic could make sure that the patient stayed below the 500 calorie limit. Here, you will be doing the program at home, without an expensive clinic to measure the food for you. There is a table that shows each of the foods and the caloric value. Once you learn how to mix and match the foods on the list and stay under 500 calories for the day, don't bother counting.

The program is not about calories, so don't substitute other 'low calorie' items in the food list. Keep below the 500, using the foods listed.

Stick to the Plan

However and whenever, you must do so. Faithfully. Eat a protein, vegetable and fruit at each meal; the bread is optional. Many people have difficulties even eating that much, so if you cut back, have at least a little of the vegetable and fruit, but take all of the protein.

Don't Substitute

 If it is not on the list, don't take it. Don't attempt any complex justifications like "well, they just didn't have this to evaluate when this was originally written" or "this has a lower glycemic index than that" or "it has no calories, so it does not count" or "this is a low calorie dish". If it is not on the list, forget it. This is not about calories, glycemic index or fiber. It is not about substitution or adjustment...on the list OK, off the list NOT OK. It's a simple rule, but often the most creative people have the hardest time with it, because they come up with any number of fascinating explanations as to why some substitution should be just fine. The original protocol expressed the same frustration, and our own studies have borne it out. Have faith; the list is complete and correct. Even if it seems boring at first, you can do anything for six weeks with results like this.

Many people express that they didn't have a problem substituting this or that, or adding some no calorie addition, but they also invariably lost less than those who stuck to the plan faithfully. What would they have lost had they stuck to the plan? There is no way to tell. However, when the same people stick to the plan in subsequent rounds, they lose more.

Another item to be careful about is minor additives in prepackaged food. Stay away from ANYTHING not on the list, and the list does not include Dextros Hydrolized anything or any other chemicals.

Don't Exercise

This is another truth that is hard to believe, as it is also contrary to conventional wisdom and belief. Normally on a very low calorie diet a person just does not have the strength to do a high-energy workout; on this program you will. Many times people report feeling great during the workout and really enjoyed having the extra energy for the first time in a long time. Then the next day they feel kitten weak, and the feeling continues for two to three days. They feel lethargic, exhausted and run down.

On this diet, there is not much exercise. No more than an hour of walking a day is really needed. People doing less still lost weight quickly. In fact, heavy work outs are not recommended. Here is what the original protocol says on the matter:

> "...the weight can temporarily increase – paradoxical though this may sound – after an exceptional physical exertion of long duration leading to a feeling of exhaustion. A game of tennis, a vigorous swim, a run, a ride on horseback or a round of golf do not have this effect; but a long trek, a day of skiing, rowing or cycling or dancing into the small hours usually result in a gain of weight on the following day, unless the patient is in perfect training. In patients coming from abroad, where they always use their cars, we often see this effect after a strenuous day of shopping on foot, sightseeing and visits to galleries and museums. Though the extra muscular effort involved does consume some additional calories, this appears to be offset by the retention of water which the tired circulation cannot at once eliminate. "

We found that we could still do the workout we were accustomed to, though maybe not quite as much of it. If the normal routine was half an hour on the Stairmaster™, 20 minutes would give the same effect. While on the diet it is not the time to increase your workout program, unless of course, you aren't doing anything at all. If you are not doing any exercise, consider taking up a little walking with the new-found energy you have. Don't go crazy with it. Don't jump into an hour long power walk...start slowly, perhaps ten minutes walking the dog, and slowly increase it as that becomes easy.

Unlike a normal low calorie diet, the body has plenty of energy on hand and that's why the initial work out is possible, and even feels good. However the next day the body needs to rebuild the muscles used during the exertions and the body puts a priority on this task. As a result, the body is not spending its energy dissolving fat for food, and the person feels like he is on a low calorie diet because the additional calories from emptying the storehouse fat have dried up. We can't change the way the body looks at its priorities, but what we can do is not ask it to choose.

So remember, exercise should be limited to a mild walk of no more than an hour a day.

Don't get me wrong, I'm a huge fan of exercise. Let it be done at the right time, though. The severely overweight person needs to reduce the fat before an exercise program has its best effect. Let's put it this way. If you wanted to build your biceps you might do some weight lifting. But if your arm was broken, the same weight lifting program that would build you up will only hurt, and probably cause more damage in the long run. The weight lifting itself is not bad, but it is not the best thing to do while injured. So let's fix the injury first. Let's reset your body's weight regulator, get you to a healthy weight and then build the program to develop muscles. One step at a time.

Don't Take Supplements

Most diets today require some sort of high-protein supplement or pills that encourage fat blocking or starch blocking or metabolism boosters that temporarily alter the body response system. This program is about getting the body to adjust itself and working with the body.

While on the program, don't take supplements. That's right; don't take extra vitamins or pills. The original protocol says not to take any medication, but before stopping any prescribed medication you **must** consult your physician. Supplements that are oil-based like cod liver oil, coconut oil, vitamin E or others that are similar must be stopped because your body is already processing a great deal of oil during the program. There is no need to burden it further. What's more, the body will have plenty of vitamins as it breaks down the storehouse fat, so there is no need for other supplements.

Prescriptions for blood pressure, water pills and diabetes medication are likely to need adjustment quickly as your body starts to change and regulate its own systems. Monitor these with your doctor carefully and adjust accordingly. Many in our study group, with their doctor's review, cut back or totally eliminated prescription medication while on the program.

True and False

No Saggy Skin

This is, understandably, a huge concern for anyone who has lost weight on a diet, or seen someone who has lost weight on a regular diet. The skin becomes saggy where the person was previously overweight. Not on this program.

Here is why: Regular diets are based on the premise that we can rob our bodies of enough calories to meet the daily demands, and the body will take the remainder from the fat stores. It does, but it only borrows them temporarily. Because the body has a long-term plan to restore the emergency reserve fat as soon as possible, it takes it from the easiest place to restore it, from inside the fat pocket. As a result, the last of the fat to be dissolved is the layer between the skin and the outer edge of the fat pocket. This does not allow the skin to retract, leaving it 'saggy'. The body will fill this in where possible with replacement fat, or sometimes the person will undergo surgery to remove the excess skin. Either way, it is not a pleasant thought for the prospective weight loss hero.

On this program however, the body is not borrowing, but rather deliberately dismantling the storehouse fat. As a result of deliberate use rather than temporary borrowing, the body takes from the outside of the fat store, between the skin and the fat, allowing the skin to retract. Because the program allows no more than 34 pounds loss in a round before a break, the body has time to adjust and complete the retraction before once again losing weight.

People who have been grossly overweight have seen the same result over and over, and are amazed that the skin retracts in a way they never have before. This is unlike any other program they have done before. Women who have had multiple children are thrilled to find that the semicircle of extra skin between the hip bones also retracts back to a flat stomach they never thought they would ever see again.

Don't Stress About Food Again

When you are done with the program, YOU ARE DONE. There is no continued counting of calories, taking supplements, or counseling programs. You will have reset the body's weight regulator, so you will maintain the new set weight. You will go back to eating what you want, when you want and not worry about weight gain. Now, that really does not seem possible until you consider that your tastes are going to change. What you craved before will be 'nice but not necessary' or you will want the taste of popcorn, but stop at a handful rather than the whole bag. The program gives you the opportunity to actually listen to your body and learn what you want. Most people reported wanting better food, because they did not want to eat as much. What they had, they wanted to be good, flavorful and rich, rather than empty calories to fill volume. When we say you will eat what you want, it is the absolute truth, but you probably won't 'want' a deep fried Twinkie. Even if you do, your body will not be hungry while it burns that off. Your weight regulator will adjust your metabolism naturally to burn off the excess and keep you at your new set correct weight. People on the program don't believe this one fully until they are ten weeks in and they see it for themselves...but accept it as a working theory for the moment.

Statements Not True on This Program

"Losing weight too fast isn't healthy and will only result in it coming back."

Well, yes, on a normal diet that would be true. This is not a diet.

Most of us are told that we should not lose more than a pound a week if we want to keep it off. This seems to be about the rate that the body can take from the storehouse fat and put it into the Normal fat processing center for consumption.

"A 500 calorie diet is dangerous!"

Yes, that is a true statement. However, this is not a 500 calorie diet. Such a diet would eat through the normal and Structural fat in the body quickly, and then start eating muscle. The body would slow down to the lowest possible activity level. The body would send out every possible signal to eat something, including being hungry all the time, being grouchy and filled with headaches and misery.

This program *does* involve eating 500 calories a day - in addition to the HCG. The HCG opens the storehouse fat doors and allows the body to take freely from there, where before it was closed off. The body takes about 2,000-3,000 calories a day from there, as a matter of fact. In effect, it is a 2,500-3,500 calorie diet, only 500 of which are going between the teeth. This allows the body to dissolve between half a pound and a full pound of fat a day.

I had a friend who started the diet, lost nine pounds the first week, and then was convinced by her next door neighbor, who was a nurse, that a 500 calorie diet was a terrible thing and should never be done. She did not have the articulation to explain that the body was using the fat to make up the calories, and the HCG made it possible to use the storehouse fat. She knew it was working; she had just lost nine pounds! But the next door neighbor scared her with all the horrible things a very low calorie diet can do to a person. Another one of the Shrinking Friends was a nurse who read up on the program and decided to give it a try. Her fellow health care professionals counseled her not to, but she had seen the results other team members were getting and forged ahead. They promised that they would "Be there to nurse her back to health." After the first round when she lost 30 pounds, they were shocked, amazed and then everyone wanted to try. It is unfortunate that those who have not read or done the diet believe they are helping by telling people how wrong such a dangerous diet is. What they are actually telling them is how wrong such a diet is, without the HCG and the full knowledge of this program.

"This is not endorsed by the American Medical Association."

HCG is approved by the FDA as a drug and is considered safe for human consumption, though the weight loss program is not currently endorsed by the AMA. However, this is the same AMA that recommended smoking for pregnant women in a day when the smoking industry was a powerful lobbyist. Enough said.

Update for the second edition: In 2012 the FDA made a crack down on Homeopathic HCG. There were several places selling water labeled HCG and encouraging people to use it on the HCG diet. Well, this is nothing more than a starvation diet if you are not using real HCG. Because HCG is an actual medication, labeling water (or HCG watered down so much that almost none remains) fell under their control, and they had it removed. Some people have mistakenly believed that this was an outlawing of the diet itself, no, it was an outlawing of the false version of the diet that some tried selling. The diet is still valid….HCG – real HCG – is still available. Unfortunately, you can still find water labeled HCG as well. Rule of thumb – if it is pre mixed particularly in a liquid form, it is not the real thing.

"You're going to be hungry all the time."

Wrong again. Because your body is dissolving fat for energy, there is little or no hunger. Nancy was funny. Before she started she was SURE that she would be hungry all the time, she had tried very low calorie diets before and been starving the whole time. We all tried to tell her, but she would not hear it. By the time she hit the second week she realized she did not want to even finish what she was supposed to eat. She lost 34 pounds, the maximum, on the first round. The program does not care if you are skeptical; it still works for you.

I'm not saying there is no desire to eat; there is, mostly because we remember wanting to eat. But there is very little or no actual hunger.

The hunger mechanism is triggered by the reduction in "normal" fat in the body; after all, this is the normal repository for day to day fuel. The first two days of the program involve fat loading. When done properly this keeps the normal fuel reserve (fat) high and never triggers the hunger response because the body goes straight to the Abnormal fat.

The program is a unique opportunity to learn the difference between 'wanting' something and 'needing' something to eat. Most people believe that they know the difference between want and need, and they probably have a very good handle on it. It is extremely difficult, however, to know - unless there is no physical need for food. Pay attention to your wants and needs during the program. This will help you to distinguish them when the program is over, and you are at the weight you want to be.

"You can't expect to overcome genetics."

Genetics did not cause you to be overweight, or even be a specific shape. Genetics may have given you a predisposition to damaging your body's weight regulator, and it probably helps dictate how your body reacts when the weight regulator is damaged. Heredity, however, has nothing to do with actually damaging the body or healing it. Think of it like breaking a bone. If your family has a history of brittle bones then you are more likely to break a bone, but genetics did not actually break the bone. The same is true with the body regulation system. You may have a greater likelihood to damage it, and may have damaged it early in life, but you don't have to keep the injury.

"You can't stay on this diet forever."

And you are not going to. This program has a beginning and an end, and a great deal of weight loss along the way. When you have lost the weight and reset the regulator, you can return to eating what you want. Fair warning, though - your wants will change. Instead of wanting to eat the entire bag of potato chips, you are likely to only pick up a handful, and push the rest away. If that does not sound like you now, you will be in for a huge surprise in six to eight weeks. The more cycles you do to lose weight, the more this seems to be the case. The thinner body does not need as many calories to function and you will have the opportunity to learn what your body is asking for rather than eating out of habit. These two items together tend to change the wants of the person who has completed the program.

Kathy finished up the program in time to get on a cruise for her anniversary. She knew she would be doing the program again, so she was not worried about what she ate or when. In fact, she says she ate everything. She put on a whole pound by the end of the two week cruise, and it fell away shortly after. Here is what she told other team members:

> "Tobi is sooo right! No need to freak out between rounds....4 weeks since the end of the
> first round, eating really well, pizza...hamburgers!!! And NO weight gain...there's no way I would have believed this!!!!!"

"There is a study that shows HCG doesn't actually do anything."

There are actually three individuals who claim to have done studies. One can't produce any records or demographic information. The other used homeopathic HCG. Some homeopathic remedies have value; however, Dr. Simeons defined a very specific strength of HCG for the program. The homeopathic version is significantly watered down, to the point that there may be no HCG left. It is, in effect, little better than water. So, the second study compared people who used water and people who used water that had once shared a room with HCG. Not surprisingly, the results were the same. Also, not surprisingly, the few people who tried it stayed on the diet only a few days and were hungry the whole time. The third did not use the food list or prohibitions about exercise and lotions and oils, and achieved similar results to those on the diet alone. We found this to be the case also, the dramatic weight loss and body reset were achieved when the exact protocol was followed, and people stalled out when they strayed from the food list or used lotions or exercised excessively. None of the others talked about the change in body shape or keeping the weight off. These are two very significant differences between this program and a weight reduction diet.

Frank, who was very impatient to start, ordered the homeopathic HCG mixture, because it would get to him quickly. He started the low calorie diet phase and found that he did lose some weight, but he was gaunt, dizzy, tired, and grumpy and after a few days he nearly passed out doing normal daily activities. By then, the actual HCG had come in, and he started the full dose HCG. He not only lost his appetite, but gained energy, and lost his weight much faster. In fact, he lost 24 pounds in three weeks. He is now down to his military weight, and stunned that it all came off of the waist and stomach. Frank was somewhat skeptical about there being a 'placebo' effect to the HCG, but now he is a living testament to just how real the HCG program is and how it makes a true difference. Not long ago I saw him at a social event and to my surprise he stripped off his shirt and exclaimed:

"I have my 1st Sergeant's body back!"

He did indeed have his active duty body and fitness he had long missed.

"It does not teach a lifestyle change, so it is not a permanent solution."

The program does not teach a lifestyle change….it just makes one. Some lifestyle changes advocate exercise; we have discussed that above. Some suggest changing the diet to healthier, fresh foods. If you don't have a taste for this, it hardly seems worth it. During the course of the program, you will eat fresh food, and after a while, it will be possible to taste the chemicals in canned and processed food. Generally, these will become undesirable. No, the program does not insist on changing what you eat for life, or how you exercise, but you are likely to anyway.

One of the basic premises is that we overeat because we are overweight, not the other way around. When the weight is reduced, the desire for food is correspondingly reduced. While reducing, the average person makes changes in what he wants to eat and how much he eats. By the time you've achieved your healthy weight, a meal that would have been normal before is no longer normal; you will be unlikely to even finish it. Many people reported that foods that they hated before now taste wonderful, flavorful and far better than they imagined.

"If this is so great, why doesn't everyone endorse it?"

The short answer is because there is no money in it. The HCG is inexpensive, because there are several manufactures and no patent on the process to develop it, so no money is to be made there. There are no long-term meetings or counseling sessions, no food programs to make money on, no gadgets to sell, no way to get rich. Why would anyone spend the money advertising and endorsing something that did not make money? This program is the ultimate grass-roots improvement process, a chance for people to take back their lives one person at a time. The only endorsement will be you, telling your friends who see you lose weight without great hardship. I recommend that when you tell your friends, you put a copy of this book in their hands. Almost invariably those that tried this from "what a friend said," without reading the details, did not do as well. There is a great deal of detail, and no room for error; get them a copy.

Side Effects

There are side effects, but they are not what you would expect on a diet. There are mental and physical changes, attitude adjustments, self esteem and perception changes. Side effects are not always negative things.

Physical Changes

I don't know when I stopped noticing my legs rub together when I walked. Not many of us really pay attention to it, because we walk all the time. On the program, when the weight is dropped, this will stop, and when it does, you will notice the difference, eventually. Pants fit better and wear less on the inside of the legs, walking is easier and cooler. The change will creep up on you, and at some point you will be startled by it, just wait.

Airline seats will get larger. I'm fairly sure every seat in every airline has been adjusted to let me fit better. We all found lots of places the gremlins went out and adjusted furniture to make it more comfortable. The airline seats were just the first ones I noticed.

Clothes shopping becomes a new experience. All too often we don't like the clothes because we look fat in them...it's not the clothes. Trying on clothes now will look better than you were expecting and the natural desire will be to buy that outfit because you look great in it...try to resist. Unless you are at your finish weight, you are going to be moving past that weight quickly and the new outfit you just got will be oversized and baggy before you make use of it. Hold out as long as you can and save up for your new wardrobe.

Your shape will change. Women end up with the classic hourglass figure; men with the V shaped chest and waist . It really does not matter what shape you were; pear, apple or watermelon, the program takes from the Abnormal fat stores and as a result, returns the person to a healthy, proportioned body. For some of us, we had never seen this shape in the mirror, and it was a surprise.

Other side effects include the change in the taste of food. The chemicals are more obvious, the food more rich, and as a result, you will find that you choose your food more carefully. You will want what tastes good.

Many dropped medications that they had been slave to for years. High blood pressure medication and heart medication in particular needed frequent adjustment or elimination all together. Other medications that were no longer needed by the team included pain medications and insulin for diabetes. There were a few cases where some specialty medications were no longer needed; it is just a matter of finding out what the body will fix on its own when it resets. Note that in the cases of dropping or modifying of prescription medications, the individual's doctor was involved. Again, consult with your physician before making any changes to prescribed drugs.

Mental Changes

I mentioned the body shape would change; this has both a physical and mental component to it. You may find it difficult to understand the new shape. This is a rather difficult concept to grasp, but you can see the difference, and still not comprehend it. For me, I knew that my waist was smaller, my legs smaller, but I did not understand until I could pull my old pants off without unbuttoning them, or I put them on and they just fell off, or I slipped on a pair of my husband's jeans, that I would not have been able to put my leg in before. If you asked me to point to someone who had my same body shape, I would be wrong, every time. It took someone else to point out similarly-shaped people. Pictures helped as well. One of the exercises I ask people to do is take a picture before you start the program. You can compare this to what you look like when you are done........even those in this book were amazed that they changed that much. Kim, a fairly-fashion conscious friend in the program realized she had to start checking the mirror every time she went out, a habit that she had stopped someplace along the line:

"Last week of the diet, I was getting dressed to go to lunch with a friend, so I chose a favorite blouse. I got dressed and, luckily, took a look in the mirror. That blouse looked TERRIBLE on me! It hung like a shapeless sack because it was 2 sizes too big! I grabbed another top and found the same thing. The third one I chose, a top that has been a little too snug for a while, looked great. The others went into the donations bag. I'm having to retrain my eye on what will fit me these days because my brain isn't yet used to seeing my body like this. Not that I'm complaining!"

Your knowledge and ability to cook will change. Because the program requires fresh food with specific ingredients without additives, preservatives or chemical flavor enhancers, the average person is going to have to do a little cooking at home. Most people began to experiment with spices and recipes and slowly became more adventurous in their cooking. Because the ingredients are limited, the beginning chef has opportunity to learn the properties of the foods better, and experiment with new techniques rather than attempting to figure out how different foods react to different processes. It is a great way to learn to cook, and some of the recipes in the back are flavor parties for the mouth.

Your desire to eat out is likely to change some as well. Because you will taste the food more, many of the commercially prepared foods will be less appealing. The up side to this change is that you are likely to spend far less eating out, and you can save that money for your new wardrobe!

Perhaps one of the most intriguing changes is the outlook to those still overweight. A great many of us all wanted to rush out and tell someone about the program, help them along, let them see how easy it was. For the first time, we get to choose our weight, and we begin to look at those who are overweight as being that way by choice rather than anything else. Ultimately, perhaps it will be by choice. For now, I'm simply making the assumption that the overweight people do not yet know how unbelievably fantastic this program is, or how they too can find the fit person inside. When you find that you just can't stop talking about how easy and well this worked, make sure you point them to where to find the book.

Emotional Changes

This program offers the unique opportunity to differentiate between want and need. I want that German chocolate cake with extra frosting, but I don't need it. We think we know the difference, but until the actual need for any kind of calories is removed, it is impossible to actually *know* the difference. It is perhaps this change that most allows a person to take a handful of pretzels and walk away from the rest of the bowl when they are done with the program.

Self esteem is probably the largest single emotional change that will occur. One of the team commented that all the 'after' pictures featured better tans. It is true - we tend to go out more, put on more revealing clothes, show off more, even, for many, go out in bikinis again. Self esteem changes as people tell us that we look great, marvel at our success, congratulate us and stand in awe of our new bodies. The more they do it, the more we are encouraged to continue, and the easier it gets to stick to the program.

Self esteem affects us in other ways as well. Most of the people noticed that their posture changed, they were taken more seriously at work, people respected them more, and they all around became more successful in public, work and private life.

One of our team members confessed that she had struggled with food all her life, she had at times been on the edge of various eating disorders. She realized on this program that she no longer had to be guilty about eating a particular food, or any food. If she put on weight, she knew how to remove it, quickly and easily. No longer was she a slave to food, and how it made her feel. She could choose her weight, and food choices or desires would not need to come into play. Others commented on the change in outlook about weight loss advertisements, realizing they no longer had any appeal, and no longer stirred feelings of guilt or inadequacy. Many interactions in the day with the TV, advertising, friends, food and so on take on a whole new very positive 'feel' to them. It is something only the person no longer a slave to watching weight can feel.

Who Should and Should Not Use the Program

Dr. Simeons referenced patients who wanted to lose as little as five pounds. The least amount lost in our group was ten pounds. Those losing so little lost it within a week; however, the minimum time to reset the hypothalamus is 21 days, and it requires that the HCG be taken for a minimum of 21 days. The HCG allows the unlimited use of Abnormal fat for fuel; however, it does not allow the body to use Normal and Structural fat for fuel. When the Abnormal fat is exhausted, the person becomes hungry, irritable and generally unpleasant. Listen to your body, it will tell you when you no longer have Abnormal fat. Anyone with more than 5-10 pounds to lose can benefit from the program.

Dr. Simeons did not address the topic of childhood obesity, possibly because it was not a significant issue 50 years ago; today, however, it is an epidemic. HCG has been used to treat immature adolescents who have failed to develop secondary sexual characteristics. Because it accelerates the maturity of sexual characteristics, it should be only be used by those who are sexually mature. The adolescent MUST consult with a physician before attempting this program.

The Program

The original protocol, as written by Dr. Simeons, does not have "Phases," however several people have broken it down into distinct phases in order to make discussion easier. The phases are Preparation, Weight Loss, Stabilization, and Ongoing. In the Preparation phase there are tasks that can be done to help set you up for success; don't skip this step. Weight Loss is the main part most people are interested in It is quick, and the results are dramatic. Stabilization is what is done between rounds to help maintain the loss and de-stress the body. In the Ongoing phase, it is all about how to keep your shape and weight forever without stressing over counting calories, while eating what you want. Don't take these last two lightly, moving through these phases is as important as losing the weight, because you want to keep it off forever, and you can - with a little effort at the beginning of these phases.

The normal person will spend about two weeks in the Preparation phase while they acquire the HCG, do research, consult with a physician if they wish and plan the food they will eat. The first round of Weight Loss lasts no more than six weeks or 34 pounds, whichever is reached first. The more diligent the person is at following the exact program, the more likely she is to get to the 34 pound mark before the six week mark. The first round of Stabilization lasts six weeks. The person who needs to lose more then goes back to the Weight Loss phase and again is limited to six weeks or 34 pounds. The next round of Stabilization is eight weeks. The Weight Loss and Stabilization phases are repeated until all the weight is gone, or until you want to stop. Then the person enters the Ongoing phase. The first two to three weeks are important to make sure the results are set for life.

Phase I – Preparation

Phase I is called the Preparation phase. If you have any concerns about your health, special medication or questions about how safe this is, consult your doctor. Increasingly, doctors are willing to prescribe the HCG for patients if they ask for it specifically. Others will point you to online pharmacies such as www.alldaychemist.com to order the HCG. All Day Chemist temporarily had to stop selling HCG because the FDA crackdown mistakenly identified them as selling Homeopathic HCG. While the FDA could not touch them directly, but they contacted VISA and VISA asked them to comply with the FDA or stop using VISA. They will get it sorted out eventually, but in the mean time, there are others such as: buyHCG123.com and rxhealthdrugs.com. The good thing about ordering from an overseas pharmacy is that it is generally less expensive than a pharmacy in the US. Federally, the law allows a 90 day supply of a drug for personal use to be purchased from an overseas pharmacy and mailed directly to you. Legal specifics may be different in your state; check your state for specific regulations. The overseas pharmacies generally do not ask for evidence of a prescription to fill the order, so you will not need access to a fax machine. A full six week round will cost about $35. If it costs much more, shop around. If it is offered from inside the US and does not require a prescription it is highly suspect, as a prescription is required if true HCG is purchased from any US-based source. DO NOT BE FOOLED BY HOMEOPATHIC HCG!!!!!

At the online pharmacy of your choice you will be presented with a wide variety of options when ordering. If mixing to take as drops under the tongue you will need 10,000 IU for each six week cycle. If mixing the HCG for injection it is only 5,000 IU for a cycle. You may wish to order more than one cycle worth to save on shipping. Figure that you will lose between 20-30 pounds in a cycle. Be sure to order one that is sent in powder form, and has a rubber stopper. The powder keeps for up to a year, and the rubber stopper is easier to open.

IU stands for "International Unit" and is used to identify a specific strength. This insures that individual manufacturers provide the same amount of medication for calculating dosages. It does not matter if you choose one 10,000 IU vial or two 5,000 IU vials, or even five 2,000 IU vials. If you are planning to mix for injections get the lower dosage vial at 1,000 IU, as this will be easier to measure.

A person who has less than 20 pounds to lose should consider doing a 'short round' of 21 days instead of 42. Actually a short round is anything over 21 days, up to a full 42 days. The minimum to reset the body is 21 days. We will get into the details of how to do a short round later. If you are doing a short round, consider purchasing in 2000 IU increments that will last 8 days each to avoid waste.

Again, plan on losing between 20-30 pounds a round. About 15% of people max out at the top weight loss in a round of 34 pounds. About 5% lose only 20 pounds. The variance depends on how much you have to lose; the heavier people will lose faster. How well you keep to the program also has an impact; even those who just can't seem to resist the occasional cheat or complete meal off the program still lose 20 pounds. Finally, it also depends on how much your body needs to reshape. There are days where no weight is lost, but a great deal of reshaping occurs. This is one of the largest differences between a weight loss program and this program. In this program, the body reshapes as well as reduces.

If ordering from an overseas pharmacy, it normally takes about two weeks for delivery.

If you are having difficulty finding it google some of the brand names and the word 'buy' such as: Corion, Hucog, Ovidac, Proficient, Fertigyn, Lupi or Sifasi. You are looking for a glass vial (preferably with a rubber stopper) with a small amount of powder. The price should be no more than 16-20 for 5000 IU (1/2 rounds worth). Shipping might be as much as $25, but it is usually a fat rate for any number of vials.

WARNING!!!!!

Do not purchase a homeopathic variety of HCG. This is extremely diluted and does not stand up to the dosing recommendations in the original protocol. There are several programs out there that are attempting to make money on the HCG program, and they promise you can lose "40 pounds in 40 days" or "100 pounds in 100 days" or "1 to 2 pounds a day," or allow you to order their product (Homeopathic HCG) for anywhere from $150 - $600 dollars. First, the program specifically says no more than 34 pounds in a round of 42 days and loss is an average of half to a full pound a day – so those making these other claims are not following the original protocol. Second, diluted HCG is never specified in the protocol – specific doses are identified. It makes you wonder how they can claim all the successes of Dr. Simeons' work, when they are not following his program. I think they are hoping you will not notice that they are referencing a different product. If they are not following the original protocol, you have to wonder whose research they are using to make these claims. I get a little steamed on this point, because this is where some of the bad press about the program comes from, particularly since those who do lose some weight because they tough out the hunger, put it back on later, and never actually reset the weight regulator.

I can't stress this point enough. There are plenty of online sites to promise you a money back guarantee for their Homeopathic HCG that works just as well as pure HCG, no waiting required! That is to say they sell you on the idea that a Mercedes™ is a really great car, look at all the wonderful things it can do, including drive 600 miles on one tank of gas! Now, buy this skateboard and see how wonderful the Mercedes™ skateboard is! Don't worry, you will be satisfied, it is just as good - it has a money back guarantee! They are all too happy to sell you something with a money back guarantee that is all but impossible to fulfill. After some heartache when it becomes clear that the skateboard does not perform as well as the Mercedes™ sports car, the attempt to follow up on the money back guarantee requires that you drive the skateboard for a full 600 miles before returning. I'm not kidding. We have had a few people fall into this trap, and it is heartbreaking to see them fail when they were so close to the solution. Take the time to get the real HCG – it is what this protocol requires.

Sites that promote the following should be avoided:

> "Lose 40 pounds in 40 days" (not according to the original protocol).
> "Proprietary formula" (Not HCG).
> "1 to 2 pounds a day" (Not according to the original protocol).
> "1x, 2x, 3x Strength" (Not HCG).
> "Our sublingual serum" (Not HCG).

"Money back guarantee" (When was the last time you found a pharmacy with a money back guarantee? And have you read the requirements to get that money back?).

If you do an internet search on "HCG diet" you will find many programs out there willing to sell you a high cost product, asking $150-$600 for watered down HCG and often a high cost group to join. This is one of those cases where the real thing is actually far less expensive.

Don't be taken in by 'special products' either. The protocol says to stop using oil-based cosmetics and lotions. The body will be moving around a great deal of oil. Even those who have had dry skin in the past did not seem to have any symptoms of that while they were on the program, even in the winter. However, there are plenty of companies out there willing to sell you protocol-friendly soaps and conditioners, even shampoos. You can buy them if you want, but it doesn't really make a difference. Almost all soaps and shampoos are 'protocol friendly'. You don't need special soaps, conditioners or shampoos. And lotions are not on the plan. Save yourself some money; no matter the hype it will not make the program faster, better or healthier. It will, however, line someone's pockets. I'd rather it stay in yours, so you can buy a copy of this book to share with a friend. ☺

Things to do While Waiting

There are plenty of things to prepare while you are waiting for your order to arrive or your appointment with your doctor.

Read the protocol
It is way too tempting to skip to the food list and mixing instructions and attempt to try the diet based on those two pages alone. Take the time to read the whole process, learn what is going on in the body, learn what to expect. Reading the protocol is the single best thing you can do to ensure your success. Don't get me wrong, you can be successful without reading the details, it is just harder...and this is about making this whole process easy. Make sure you know what is on the food list, detailed in the Phase II section, and stock up on the ones you like.

Read the directions carefully on how to progress through the diet. *DO NOT SKIP THIS STEP.* It is important to understand what you are going to be doing and when. There is no room for variation in this program. The plan is not difficult to follow, but it is precise. Unlike most diets, you will immediately stall if something is done contrary to the plan. Depending on what is done, weight can even be gained. While this may not seem like a great deal at first, it is lost time. Every day that is lost from falling off the plan is a day taken from the 40 days you can stay on the HCG in a round. After the 40 days a person must take a break to prevent developing immunity to the HCG. In effect, when someone goes off the diet, it is not just one day longer before they reach the weight they want, it might be more than six weeks because they must wait to start another round. Most people decide in the first maintenance round that they don't want to cheat on the program again, because they don't want to wait to reach their goal. We will discuss this in greater detail later.

Clean out the kitchen
If you live alone, or if everyone in the house is on the plan, put away everything you can't have on the diet. If you live with others, clear out a shelf in the fridge just for you. It's easier not to graze on forbidden food if you don't have any in sight.

Print out the food list and keep a copy on the fridge
Knowing what you can and can't have is helpful for quick meal plans. The list is easy to remember, and in short order you won't need it. But in the beginning, take the precaution so you know what is allowed.

Take 'Before' measurements and pictures
Most people don't want to do this part, but do it. You will NEVER be this size again; you will never be able to take this picture again. You don't have to share it, you don't have to show it to anyone, but when you want to compare after your first round, you can't ever go back and recapture it. In addition, there will be days when the loss seems to stall or slow down, these are times that your body is changing shape, and you are retaining extra water to move around the fat and waste. Measurements will help keep you motivated. I know you don't

want to, but do it, you won't regret it, and it won't cost you anything but a few minutes of time. When taking the picture, wear clothes that "fit" in each stage, and are similar in color and type (it will make the comparison easier to see). Some people chose the same form fitting workout clothes in progressively smaller sizes to show the difference. Clothes that show as much skin as you are willing to show are best; this will allow you to see bulges and rolls disappear. Remember, you don't have to share these, but they will be absolutely inspirational to others when you can show the comparison. Most people hardly believe the change when the photos are side by side, and the ones who did not take them usually regret that decision.

For measurements, take:

- Neck
- Upper arm
- Under the arms, measured around the body
- Women: just under the bust. Men: Chest
- Waist
- Abdomen
- Hips
- Middle of the thigh
- Calf

Consider making a spreadsheet to track your weekly loss. The Fat2Fab website has a spreadsheet example to use for tracking that calculates weekly and total loss.

Clean out your spice cabinet

Replace the old spices. Spices become an important part of the program. Your taste buds will come alive again once they are not inundated with fast food, and processed or packaged food with additives. It's hard to describe, but spices take on a whole new impact. Get fresh ones where you can.

Track your water consumption

Find a way to measure how much water you drink in a day. Half a gallon to a full gallon of water is essential. The original protocol says half a gallon; our test group found that a full gallon gave better results. Fill up water bottles that equal a gallon in the morning, and make sure you sip at them all day. You can also place tape on the bottle and use a marker to note each empty/refill. Finding a way to track your consumption throughout the day will help you stay on track and keep you from trying to guzzle it all down at once at the end of the day.

Required Equipment

Small kitchen scale
Because a good part of the success of the program is based on eating exactly what is described, it is important to weigh the protein accurately. One protein portion is 3.5 ounces of uncooked meat, or 100 grams. An accurate digital kitchen scale is probably the single most important piece of equipment you will need. If you can't get a digital one, a spring one will do, but GET A SCALE. Digital scales range in price from $5 to $50 and the average is around $15.

A digital bathroom scale
This is by far the second most important piece of equipment. One of the team members did it with an accurate shipping scale at work, but I don't recommend it. The protocol asks you to weigh yourself every morning after going to the bathroom. Any small variation in loss can quickly be examined and corrected, if needed. It's also exciting to race to the scale in the morning to see how much you've lost. When is the last time you did that? A digital bathroom scale will run from $15 to $50. You don't need one that measures everything from water ratio, bone mass or anything else other than weight. Digital is better because you will see the loss in clear increments. It is also rather cool to see your body fat percentage drop as well. This is empirical proof that you are losing fat, not muscle.

Totally Optional Equipment

Hand vacuum sealer
These are easily available at the supermarket next to the plastic wrap and resalable plastic sandwich bags. Armed with the vacuum sealer and a few freezer bags, it will be easy to make, measure and store

quick meals for easy preparation. Again, it is not required, but it makes it easier to freeze and refreeze foods without freezer burn.

Food dryer
This is not required, but can make some things fun. Cucumbers salted and dried make a fun substitute for chips...apple peels dried are a chewy and flavorful snack, you might even try drying other items when you discover how fun it can be.

Small blender
This is for quick purees. I found that pureeing a half an onion and chopping the other half for a soup thickens up the end result and makes the end product much more flavorful.

CO2 unit
Totally unneeded, frivolous $30 product, but lots of fun. WWW.fizzgiz.com will lead you to a quick Co2 unit that can turn ordinary water into soda water and there is always the SodaStream©. Mix the water with a little flavored Sweet Leaf™ sugar substitute in Root Beer or Vanilla Cream flavor and Voila! Instant soda pop! This is great for people who just can't give up sodas.

SweetLeaf™ flavor drops
Absolutely not required, however it makes drinking lots of water far more interesting. They come in fun flavors like Chocolate Raspberry, Orange Soda, English Toffee, Hazelnut, Berry, Vanilla Cream and so on. It is available online for about $9 a bottle, or in many health food stores for about $15 a bottle. Look for Liquid Stevia by SweetLeaf™.

Preparing Meals
Preparation is the key to success. It is way too easy to attempt to justify a 'little' cheat when you don't have a meal handy. When a meal on the plan is only a few minutes away, it is so much easier to stay on track. Consider preparing several of these meals in advance and freezing them to keep you on track. This is where the hand vacuum sealer comes in handy.

Burgers
Make up a batch of Spiced Burgers (recipe included in the back) in chicken or beef, form into measured patties and separate with two

sheets of wax paper between each and freeze. Lots of meals can be made with the premeasured patties.

Meatballs
The recipe in the back makes a tasty meatball. Make sure to form them in more or less uniform size so that the same number will make the required serving. Freeze them in the same bag and take out the number you need for a recipe.

Baked Apples and Apple Sauce
This is an absolutely wonderful recipe that we use on or off the protocol, make extra and freeze them in half cup containers for a quick desert. Put a serving in a blender and puree for a fantastic applesauce; one serving fits in a half-cup container. **Warning**! This is not the same as a commercial Applesauce! Store-bought Applesauce has preservatives that don't belong in you for this program!

Soup Stock
Make a gallon to start (recipe included) and store in a gallon jug in the fridge. Pull it out for a quick and flavorful base to many of the soup recipes in the back.

Phase II – Rapid Weight Loss

Mixing and Taking the HCG

If you are mixing your own HCG from the overseas pharmacy, the package will come with sterile water. This is normally used for injections, but can be used for the sublingual mixing.

For drops under the tongue

You will need a solution of 1 part water and 1 part vodka. Some people have replaced the vodka with vitamin B5 or even 5-Hour Energy™. You will also need a 1ML syringe (no needle needed), a 10ML syringe is handy, but not required, and an eyedropper bottle with a screw-on cap (available in most health food stores) that can hold the complete mixture. For each 1,000IU you will need a bottle that can hold 2ML of fluid.

Some pharmacies will give these items away for mixing solutions, or administering children's medicine. The 1ML syringe holds a very small amount of fluid, and it is important to measure this accurately. Make sure you ask for a syringe, not a hypodermic – the syringe is used for measuring, a hypodermic is used for taking shots. Some states, in an effort to cut down on drug trafficking, limit the sale or distribution of hypodermics. You don't need them thinking you are a druggie...and you don't actually need a hypodermic, just the measuring body of the syringe. Make sure to refrigerate the HCG after mixing to ensure a six week shelf life.

- Mix roughly half distilled water (some often comes in the package) and half vodka or vitamin B5 complex. If you have neither, using just distilled water will work fine, though it may be harder to feel the mixture under your tongue.

- Pull off the hard plastic cap on the top of the bottle of HCG, exposing the rubber stopper.

- Cut off the aluminum band that circles the top of the bottle. This may be difficult.

- Carefully pry off the rubber stopper. Inside is a fine white powder; this is the concentrated HCG.

- Fill the 1ML syringe with the mixed fluid, and put in the small vial.

- Put the stopper back on and tip the vial gently to mix, do not shake. This will make sure the water mixture touches and dissolves the powder.

- Put one more ML in the vial and pour the mixture into the larger eyedropper bottle.

- Continue carefully measuring the fluid mixture and adding to the eyedropper bottle until you have added 2ML for each 1,000IU. For 5000IU vials, this would be 10ML of fluid.

- This will make a mixture that will equal 125IU's in .25 ml of solution. Measure out .25ML and count how many drops it takes (probably 6 or so) for your eye dropper.

- Take this many drops under your tongue twice a day in order to get a full dose sublingually (under the tongue). All drops can be taken at once, if it is more coinvent for your schedule.

For Injections

The protocol indicates 125IU's should be administered daily, once a day. To mix for subcutaneous (under the skin) injections:

- Pull the hard plastic lid off of the HCG bottle and wipe with alcohol. Do not remove the aluminum ring or stopper; you will be pushing the needle through the rubber stopper.

- Fill a syringe with air and pierce the plastic vial full of sterile water with the syringe needle, and inject it with air......this creates a positive pressure inside the bottle.

- Withdraw 1ml of sterile water and inject into the HCG vial.

- Withdraw 1ml of air from the HCG vial to make room for additional water.

- Repeat steps 2 and 3. You now have 2 ml of fluid in the small, sealed HCG vial. The strength of this solution and how much you need to take is dependent on how many IU's were in the original bottle.   A 1,000IU vial will yield 8 injections of .25 ml (125IU per injection). A 2,000IU vial will yield 16 injections of .125 ml (125IU per injection). Bottles with 5,000IU in them require such a small measurement they are not recommended for using for injections.

Consult with your physician on the best way to administer injections. The insulin needles are quite small and can barely be felt, and are given subdurally (under the skin) or intramuscularly (in a muscle).

The first two days
The first two days of taking HCG involves 'Fat Loading.' This is done by eating fat, as much as you can for the first two days, while taking the drops. This helps ensure that the body has enough Normal fat and will help prevent hunger as the body switches over to the storehouse fat. It also takes about two days to open the storehouse fat door. It will also take two days to close the doors at the end of the cycle, and this is why you will continue the menu restriction two days after stopping the drops.

Fat does not equal carbohydrates, nor does fat loading mean 'eat anything you want.' That is to say, a slice of bread with butter is nice, but use the bread only as a vehicle for the fat. It is far better to fat load with cream, butter, nuts, cheese, ice cream, peanut butter and fatty meats (pepperoni, sausage, very fatty steak - in other words, leave the fat attached) rather than breads, potatoes and rice. The object here is to stock up on the 'normal' fat in the body so that your hunger response is not triggered. Remember – fat, not fattening foods, for the first two days of taking the drops.

A good fat loading day would look like:
Breakfast: bacon, sausage and a three cheese omelet
Morning snack: Cheese on crackers
Lunch: Fried Hamburger or even two, no bun, French fries,
Afternoon Snack: Potato Chips (not baked) with sour cream dip, lots of it
Dinner: Italian bread and olive oil for dipping, Alfredo sauce with a little fettuccini and cheesy garlic bread
Desert: Cheese Cake
Late night snack: Ice Cream and Oreos

It sounds impossible to eat that much fat in a day, but try. Proper fat loading will prevent being grumpy or hungry as your body makes the switch to using the fat stores.

The first week
The first week is usually the hardest, because a whole new routine needs to be developed. First thing in the morning, go to the bathroom, and weigh yourself. Record that loss. Some find it helpful to keep a food log and a record of what they lost every day to help determine which foods help lose more and which are not as effective. If you are doing this, be sure to check foods up to two days back from a low loss day to spot a trend.

Take the drops first thing in the morning and follow the food program throughout the day.

Meals and What to Eat

It is absolutely vital that the person who is preparing meals understand the restrictions associated with the food list. In the course of a day no more than 500 calories are to be consumed. The body is getting plenty of nutrition by making up the difference in what it needs by taking it from the storehouse fat. There are no additives, no cooking oils, no canned, bottled, packaged or premade food (other than what you make yourself). You will, in fact, have to cook. It can be easy, but you will have to do it to ensure the purity of what you are eating in order to reset the system.

For those cooking for others while on the program, even the smallest of tastes of a food not on the plan can derail the program. Don't taste other foods, don't sample, and don't test. If it is not on the list and included in your meal that day, don't eat it.

From the original Protocol from Dr. Simeons (additions in parenthesis):

"**BREAKFAST**:
- Tea or coffee in any quantity without sugar. Only one tablespoonful of milk allowed in 24 hours. (SweetLeaf™ may be used.)

LUNCH:
- 100 grams (3.5 oz) of veal, beef, chicken breast, fresh white fish (excluding tuna, herring, mackerel, salmon and eel which have too high a fat content), lobster, crab (not crab substitute), or shrimp. All visible fat must be carefully removed before cooking, and the meat must be weighed raw. It must be boiled or grilled without additional fat. Salmon, eel, tuna, herring, dried or pickled fish are not allowed. The chicken breast must be removed from the bird.
- One type of vegetable *only*, to be chosen from the following: spinach, chard, chicory, beet-greens, green salad, tomatoes, celery, fennel, onions, red radishes, cucumbers, asparagus, cabbage.
- One breadstick (grissini) or Melba toast.
- An apple or a handful of strawberries or one half grapefruit.

DINNER: Same four choices as lunch.

ADDITIONAL TIPS FOR SUCCESS:

- The juice of one lemon daily is allowed for all purposes. Not bottled lemon juice.
- Salt, pepper, vinegar, and all spices are allowed for seasoning but no oil, butter or dressings.
- Tea, coffee, water or mineral water are the only drinks allowed, but they may be taken in any quantity and at all times. A person should drink at least two liters of water a day, and a gallon of fluid a day is desirable – and worked better for most team members.
- The fruit or breadstick may be eaten between meals instead of with lunch or dinner.
- No more than the four items listed for lunch and dinner may be eaten at one meal.
- No cosmetics or vitamins other than lipstick, eyebrow pencil and powder may be used. This includes hand and facial lotions. The body is processing a great deal of oil and adding it to the skin will only require the body to work harder to process these oils as well. Your body while dissolving the fat will be using the vitamins previously stored there.
- You may break up the two meals; however, you cannot have two of the same type of item in a single meal. That is to say, you can't have both breadsticks or both pieces of fruit in the same meal.
- You cannot save food from one day to use the next day.
- You cannot substitute a fruit for another breadstick or anything else on the plan. Select one from each list of items, no more. One apple of any size is acceptable - two small apples, even if they are the same weight as the large one, are not.
- If in the US, consider skipping beef, as it is fattier than most European beef. Leaner meat is better.
- Don't exercise more than a mild half hour walk twice a day. You may feel like you have extra energy but using it in exercise will cause a stall and a feeling of extreme lethargy for three days. Bailing hay in the sun for three

hours is actually exercise (really, we had someone do that).

- Never exceed 500 calories. While sticking to the list is the most important aspect, staying under 500 calories is vital for the best results. The original program was conducted at an in-house hospital, where portions were controlled. It is completely possible to eat enough of a vegetable to exceed 500 calories; don't. Below is a list of the foods on the list, and the caloric count for a 100 gram portion. Make sure to stay under the limit for best results.
- Although it does not mention it in the original protocol, except indirectly, those who drank coffee and tea (in addition to at least 64 oz of water) felt that they lost more.

Food		Calories in 100 grams
Beef		139
Chicken		110
Cockles		50
Cod		100
Crab		110
Haddock		110
Lobster		100
Mussels		90
Prawns		100
Trout		100
Veal		105
Shrimp		105
Apple		44
Grapefruit		32
Strawberry		30
Tomatoes		20
Asparagus		20
Beet Greens		21
Cabbage		20
Chard		19
Celery		10
Chicory		24
Cucumber		10
Fennel		31
Leek		20
Lettuce		15
Onion		18
Radish		16
Red Onion		33
Spring Onion		25
Spinach		8
Tomatoes		20
Melba Toast		15
Grissini		11

No variations are to be introduced to the food list. All things not listed are forbidden. The meat must be measured each time. Even though some foods have less calories or less fat, if they are not on the list, they are not allowed. One of the controversial items is turkey. It was not on the original list, and has less fat than chicken breasts. Calories and fat however are not the only consideration in the program. Some items with fewer calories do not have the same composition, nor do they react the same way in the program. Peppers, okra, artichokes and pears are examples of this. Dr. Simeons does say "that chicken breast does not mean the breast of any other fowl, nor does it mean a wing or drumstick." For best results, STICK TO THE PLAN. The program works, no matter if the person is "a small elderly lady of leisure or a hard working muscular giant. Under the effect of HCG the obese body is always able to obtain all calories it needs from the Abnormal fat deposits, regardless of whether it uses up 1,500 or 4,000 a day" according to Dr. Simeons' original report.

Some people have difficulty finding the breadsticks. They are usually found in the cracker isle of the supermarket. The individual sticks are about ten inches long and a quarter of an inch wide, and have a total of 10-20 calories each. The rosemary flavored ones have no additional calories, but some do, be sure to read the label. You can buy them on Amazon.com if you can't find them anywhere else. Here is a picture of one brand:

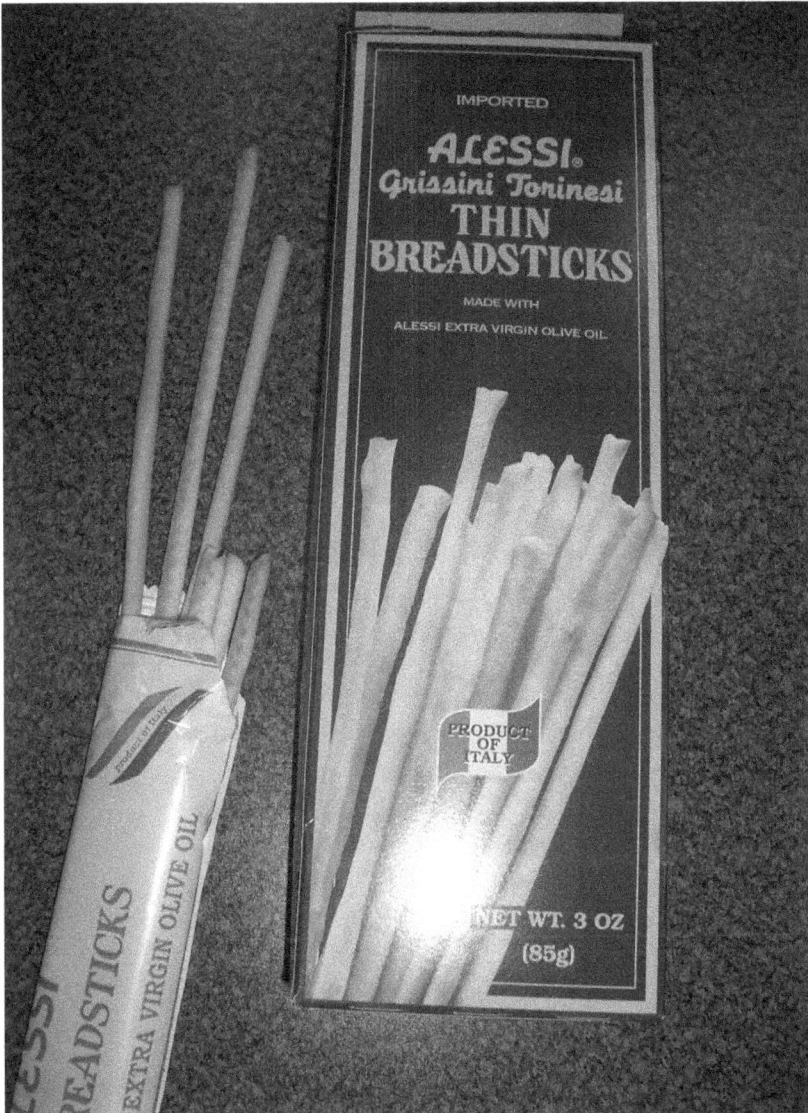

When selecting a Melba Toast option, make sure that the toast does not exceed 10-15 calories. One of the common places people get derailed is when they have a larger piece than allowed. You are allowed 1 stick pictured above, or 1 Melba Toast. Skipping this bread option is just fine.

For the vegetarian:

Strict vegetarians pose a problem. 100 grams (3.5 oz) of cottage cheese from nonfat or skimmed milk, or 8 ounces of nonfat milk can be used as a protein serving. All other choices are to be the same as the standard plan. Vegetarians do seem to lose weight more slowly.

These are not acceptable cheats

These are some of the excuses and justifications I've heard for altering the plan. The plan has no alterations. Dr. Simeons points out that 'All things not listed are forbidden.' Some people, however, just have to have something in addition, and they have an amazing array of excuses to justify them. I'm not kidding; I've heard every one of these. Just for the record – not one of them is acceptable.

"Well, I use turkey, because it is just like chicken........when the original protocol was written turkey was not that readily available, so it was not on the list."

Turkey is not chicken breast. Calories and fat are not the only items for consideration. The argument that turkey was not readily available is possible; however there was extensive work and research done to create the list. They checked artichokes and okra in Italy; they probably looked at turkey as well.

"Turkey bcon is fine, it's low in fat and it's just turkey."

Let's look at the ingredients in Turkey Bacon...wait, we don't have to...not one of them is on the list.

"I use imitation crab, it is just pollack, that's a white fish, and that's allowed."

Well, Pollock is indeed an acceptable fish...however imitation crab also has starch and other chemicals that are not on the list. The starch addition is particularly bad. Skip this one and use real crab instead.

"I'm just licking the outside of the Doritos™ - that's just spices."

Not exactly. While there are plenty of spices, there are also a great many chemicals in the tasty spice coating , including MSG in most varieties. MSG is most definitely not on the list of acceptable foods, neither are the other preservatives and colorants.

"I had a peach the other day, because it was so hard, it was just like an apple."

No. It does not matter how hard that peach is, it is just not an apple. Really. The program specifies particular foods in particular quantities. This is not just for counting calories. The specific items on the list are foods that will help reset the system. Substituting items, even if they have the same calories, does not help with resetting the hypothalamus. Keep in mind, the end goal is to reset the body's regulator for weight, not just lose the weight.

"I used fat free Parmesan cheese as my milk for the day. It's fine, it's fat free."

Um, no. Cheese of any kind is not on the list. Let's take a look at the fat free parmesan cheese container…. Which of the ingredients is not on the food list?…that would be ALL OF THEM.

"It said fat free…..so it should be ok."

While the program does take out extra fat, that is not all that the food list is concerned with. This food list is designed to give specific nutrients in specific quantities. Adding more does not help, substituting does not help.

"A cup of dried apple is the same as a cup of fresh."

No. An apple has about 65-75 calories, a cup of dried apples has over 200. Likewise, one apple of any size is not the same as several apples. On the program you can have an apple of any size, and there are some very big ones out there if you are feeling hungry. But two small ones are not the same nutritionally. The program specifies ONE per meal.

"When the protocol was written, you could only get tuna packed in oil, and that's why it is not on the list."

No, tuna is a fatty fish. Not all fish are created equal, some are fattier than others, and not all are acceptable on the program. The fatty fish are not acceptable. These include salmon of any type, tuna, mackerel, herring, sardines, orange roughy and trout. There is an interesting note on tuna packed in water though…the packing process actually takes out the oil in the cooking. For some, this is a reasonable substitute, particularly because it comes in 3 ounce packs that open with a pull tab. This is a far better choice than eating out or lunchmeat…but is still not on the food list.

"I just have my lunch and dinner breadsticks together."

How hard is it to count to "one"? The program specifies ONE breadstick in a meal. If you skip one in a meal, that's fine, but it does not mean that you can add it into the next meal or the next day. This goes for anything skipped in a meal. It cannot be added to the next meal.

"I used these no carb/no calorie noodles – that should be fine – they don't have any calories."

No, if the body is attempting to digest a no calorie fiber food, it is not dissolving fat. Give your body a chance to take away the fat. Stick to the food list, don't try to adjust it, it is only six weeks. For results like this you can tolerate a limited food choice.

It's your choice

All justifications aside, you can make your own choices. None of these are recommended for those who want to make the most of the program and lose as quickly as possible. Sometimes, however, we just can't stick to the program for whatever reason. Maybe it was a client lunch, or your sister's wedding cake……whatever it was, here is what you can expect:

Eat something not on the plan: Lose less than you would have. You may still lose the next morning, but instead of losing a pound, you might only lose .2 pound - even if the thing you ate weighs much less. The body will need to retain more water to process the additional nutrients, fat and carbs. While the body is processing this, it is not processing fat.

Eat a whole meal not on the plan: Lose three days of progress. The stall may not show up the next morning; in fact, it may not show up for two days. More likely than not though, there will be a stall, or a slow down at the very least of up to three days for a single meal.

Exercise beyond an easy walk: Temporarily stall while the body works out the additional toxins and retains water to process them. Should the workout be so strenuous as to require muscle to be rebuilt the body may actually cannibalize muscle for energy instead of rebuilding it to save efficiency. Just don't do this if you can help it.

Tips on sticking to the plan

Any deviation from the eating plan will cause a slowdown in loss. Every once and again someone insists that they were very good about staying on the program, and were disappointed that they only lost 20 pounds when those around them lost 25 or 30 or even 34 pounds in the same six weeks. Then they discuss that mixing vegetables is ok, or eating the new 'no calorie' noodles is ok, or eating turkey or tuna is fine, they did it and still lost. Yes, they still lost, however for the best results, stick exactly to the plan.

Some people don't understand that any deviation, even if it is an ounce or two, can cause several ounces to register on the scale. Take salt as an example. The body will only tolerate salt at a strength of 1 teaspoon in one liter of water. If you increased your salt intake by a teaspoon, you would gain almost two pounds to process it. While this effect is always true for salt, it is also true for all foods while taking HCG. When the program is done, the body does not retain the extra water to process additional food.

Some things you can do to break up the food, or eat more often:

- Lettuce Leaf Crunch; if you had lettuce at lunch take a leaf or two of Romaine, wet it with water and shake off the excess. Dust it with garlic salt and dill for a savory crunch snack.

- Eat an apple for a late afternoon snack, or a breadstick and an apple for breakfast.
- Keep an apple with you when you go out. A quick apple snack is far better than grabbing a meal on the road and falling off the plan. Make sure to take this off your total of two fruits for the day.
- Consider splitting a meal in half to make mini meals during the day if you worry about eating often enough. This does not seem to be satisfying for many people, as the smaller meals are not as filling.
- You can have as much of the vegetable as you wish. Crunch on more lettuce or celery or whatever the vegetable was that you had with your meal.

Trouble Shooting

- Hunger associated to the first week is usually an indication that there was not enough fat taken in on the first two days. The protocol talks about 'forcing' food, and that really is what it comes down to. Eat as much of the fatty foods as you can.
- Dizzy – not drinking enough water. A MINIMUM of a half gallon is needed, more is better – at least a gallon a day is desirable.
- Avoid diet drinks, they are loaded with chemicals that the body has to process, if it is processing those items, it is not dissolving fat.
- Avoid lotions. Your skin is an organ and your body absorbs the oils in a lotion. If it is processing these oils and chemicals, it is not dissolving fat.
- No gum or mints. Again, they have extra chemicals. It is not the weight of the chemical that will add weight; it is that your body takes time and energy away from eliminating the fat to deal with them.
- Avoid restaurant food wherever possible. They use additives to make it tastier, and again, you don't want to distract your body from dissolving the actual fat store.

- It is always 100g of PRECOOKED food. Cooking removes water and weight from foods.
- For some, it does not matter, but others may be slowed down by food choices;
  - Don't eat the same protein, or meal twice in a row,
  - Don't mix vegetables,
  - Skip American beef or at least take the leanest cut and use it sparingly
  - Avoid saccharin or aspartame

Stalls and fluctuations in weight loss

The first week often has the largest loss, however it slows down to 'one pound or somewhat less per day' according to the original protocol. Men usually lose regularly at that rate. Women can be somewhat more irregular in their loss. The most usual reason is that the body is busy rearranging fat deposits and dissolving solids, and needs the extra water to do so. Sometimes a person feels a particular area to be 'squishy' and realizes that is the next area to show loss. When a person keeps to the plan flawlessly but still does not show loss she is more likely to be showing a rapid change in inches. Hang in there, in a few days the loss will pick up.

Other predictable reasons for a stall:

- Toward the end of the round there can often be a stall for a day or two, as the body starts to compensate for the HCG. It is why the program is only 42 days before a break.
- There is also a plateau which can last 4-6 days, and happens most often, if it happens at all, in the second half of a full course. This happens as the body reorganizes.
- The next type of stall can last up to 10-14 days. This is usually because at some point you have been at that weight for an extended amount of time. This too shall pass. Keep to the plan.
- Women may stall a few days before menstruation, and some will stall when ovulating. These stalls last only a couple of days. Oral contraceptives may still be used during this program.

Bodily elimination

Expect to urinate more often, sometimes several times a night as your body dissolves fat and uses the water to flush it out of the system. Do not reduce your water intake to less than half a gallon a day; drink at least a gallon a day if you can. The water is the only way for your body to eliminate the waste product from breaking down the fat. Time and again the most successful people are the ones that drink a gallon a day.

Another side effect is a reduced need for bowel movements. A person can go three to four days without one on this program normally. If the person is very worried about this a suppository may be used, but never an oral laxative, as this causes the body to work too hard to eliminate the drug.

The last two days

The last two days stop taking the drops, but continue eating from the food list for those two days. Record the weight you were the last morning you took the drops. This is your new set weight; however, you must continue the food restriction for the next two days. While the storehouse fat doors are open, fat moves freely out of the storehouse, but it is a two way door. Any extra fat that the body has will be immediately returned to the storehouse while the door is open. You are almost there, but stick to the plan for two more days.

Phase III – Between Rounds

The first two weeks after finishing Phase II involve a slow reintegration of starches and sweets. Sweets are easy to identify: candy, soda, sugar, etc. Starches are easiest to identify as items that are near impossible to clean once they dry on a pot, such as mashed potatoes, oatmeal, rice, bread and cake batter (cakes and other flour items). If you dread cleaning it off a dried pot, it is probably a starch. Other starches include corn, potatoes and flour-based items. This does not mean you have to swear off all sugar and starch for two weeks, it just means you should not make a meal of spaghetti and garlic bread followed by chocolate cake. Eat sugar and starch sparingly, and weigh yourself every morning. Cut back on them if you see the weight creep back on.

Make sure you continue to drink water. You are already in the habit of it at this point, and it is good for you, so you might as well continue.

For the first two weeks your weight may fluctuate a little. This happens while your body is sorting out its new weight, eliminating and reestablishing your water balance, and figuring out how to maintain your new set weight. If you ever weigh in and find that you have gained more than two pounds, even just a little, from the last day that you took drops, do a 'Steak Day.' A Steak Day is done by having only coffee, tea or water throughout the day, and the largest steak you can enjoy with only a tomato as an optional vegetable. You will find that you have returned to the set weight or very close to it by morning.

Oddly, if you have lost more than two pounds, do a steak day as well. You may be tempted to just be happy with losing more, but don't fall for the trap. If you have lost more than two, your body is most likely taking out Normal fat, and will resupply it with what it lost and then some when you are eating normally again. Stick to the plan.....your progress has been great so far, go the extra step to make sure you keep it.

You may also feel a little off when it comes to moving, especially if you took off the full 34 pounds. Most say it is not exactly 'weakness' but rather that it just takes more to move. This happens when the fat is removed from between the muscles. In a few days the muscles will tighten up and the sensation will go away. Many, very active people, reported having to relearn how to move now that they weighed so much less. Don't worry, your body adapts very quickly and will generally faster and stronger than before. Remember, you've had the muscle to move that extra weight around, the muscle stayed, just the fat left, and now you have extra muscle power to spare.

Phase IV – Going forward

Once the body has stabilized after the last round of loss, take inventory. You have a new body; listen to it. Most found that they no longer wanted junk food, or if they did, they walked away after only a handful. In most cases it was remembering that they liked something, and when they tasted it, the 'something' was no longer what they wanted. Most found that they liked the taste of food better when cooked at home, and they began to taste the chemicals in fast food more. As a result, it became easier to keep the weight off, because they were listening to their bodies and eating what they wanted, rather than eating out of habit.

Should your weight increase more than two pounds from your last dosing weight, do a Steak Day. The weight will drop again. If that is not an option, eat lightly, and skip the extra cream in the latte to let your body settle back down to where it wants to be. Several people noticed that when they ate carbs their body temperature went up as if to burn it off, and they stayed the same weight. This is not uncommon. The body should naturally adjust metabolism to stay at the new set weight. It can be overwhelmed, of course, by several days of overeating, but it will attempt to return.

If the weight goes up and stays up, for over a month, even after responsible eating only when hungry, consider another round, or even a mini round. We have seen, and the protocol mentions, people who have taken off as little as 5 pounds. In these cases, the HCG must be given for a MINIMUM of 21 days in order to reset the hypothalamus. If the weight loss goal is achieved before 21 days, then increase the calories slightly, still staying away from heavy carbs until the 21 day mark is achieved. Then follow the stabilization process.

One of our weight loss team noted that her attitude toward food had changed., Because it could never stick to her again, she did not have to feel guilty about eating anything. She knew it would come off. Even if it did not she knew she could easily lose more by going on another round of the program.

Where to Stop

We all chose a goal weight to start with, but that is different than finding your ideal end weight. One of the most amazing things is that the body shape changes. As a result, most of us don't really know what we should look like, or weigh at our ideal stopping point. Over and over again the test group asked, "When do you know when to stop and just be happy with the new you?"

The truth is, if you are happy with you, it is the best thing there is. If you are happy with you, but are interested in losing more, go for it...the program is self-limiting, it will not let you lose anything but the abnormal fat. You will know that you have reached the end of the Abnormal fat loss when you are ravenously hungry and grumpy. Those who tried to use this diet to take off a few "vanity" pounds found themselves there very quickly, and it becomes obvious. You will not feel the upbeat, positive outlook you had been feeling.

But the question remains, how do you know if you should start another round? Strip and stand in front of the mirror. Are there bulges you would like to get rid of? Is there cellulite? "Orange Peel" skin? All of those can go away if you like, and you know how to do it now.

Several people, feeling 50-75 pounds lighter, were ecstatic to stop there and believed they were where they wanted to be. Great! In about six months they realized that they were at a weight that they never thought they would see again, and were very happy with that, but they were still overweight. Many started another round and continued to lose well past what they ever dreamed, and ended up at a weight their doctor would be proud of –incidentally, they are proud of it too. I did not expect to lose more than 30 pounds, which was the weight at which I had always felt most healthy. It was the weight that my best diet and exercise plan had been able to get me to. It was a weight I did not think I could ever get past. I ultimately dropped twice that and ended up with a weight that I had not had since my early twenties and a shape I'm not sure I've ever had. It's an adventure, there is a good chance you have never been here before – see where it takes you.

I recommend going to the zoo, or maybe the amusement park. Don't laugh, there is a reason really. One of the downsides of losing weight and changing shape is that your conceptualization of your body is now probably wrong. After all, you have had this body for years, you know it well, and it does not normally change this quickly or this drastically. Some of us largely just did not care, but most of us realized that we could not tell what we looked like anymore. A few things will help. First, put your before and after pictures side by side. Your first thought may be that the photo was doctored or that it was a different person...no, that's you. Next, take a friend and a camera with you to the park. Find someone that you think your new body looks like, and have your friend check you. Most likely, you have picked someone too large (we all did). When your friend finds someone they are sure is more like you, fix that in your mind, and see if they won't let you take a picture of the two of you together. Explain to them what you are doing and why, and ask, the worst they could do is say no. If that bothers you, complement their shoes, pants pattern or cut, hair color – whatever, and ask if you can take a picture with them so you can remember it. Most people will be flattered. The idea here is to get you to see yourself side by side to compare shapes and size. Pictures are extremely helpful for this.

Some places to start looking at a finish weight actually come from those impossible height/weight tables. I'll show and explain a few here, but they all have flaws. The most important thing to remember is that they are averages, and the creator of the table has never actually met you. Use them as a place to start; the ultimate judge of how you look, however, is between you and your mirror.

Military height/weight tables

Military tables seem to be the most standard for the average healthy person. They allow for a certain amount of muscle and are reasonably achievable for most. The tables are broken down by age and gender; however they make no allowance for frame size.

While some of us have used 'big boned' as an excuse to be overweight, there is some truth to the concept. The MetLife table attempts to take frame size into consideration, but more on that table later.

To read this table, weigh yourself wearing as little as possible and measure height in bare feet. Convert the height to inches, for example 5' 10" is 70 inches, and match that on the correct gender chart down the left side. Read across the top for the age bracket. Where the two lines meet is a top end weight.   The first column has a minimal weight the Army does not consider it healthy to be lower than.

ARMY Male Height/Weight Chart

HEIGHT IN INCHES	MINIMUM WEIGHT	MAX WEIGHT AGE 17 - 20	MAX WEIGHT AGE 21 - 27	MAX WEIGHT AGE 28 - 39	MAX WEIGHT AGE 40 +
58	91				
59	94				
60	97	132	136	139	141
61	100	136	140	144	146
62	104	141	144	148	150
63	107	145	149	153	155
64	110	150	154	158	160
65	114	155	159	163	165
66	117	160	163	168	170
67	121	165	169	174	178
68	125	170	174	179	181
69	128	175	179	184	186
70	132	180	185	189	192
71	136	185	189	194	197
72	140	190	195	200	203
73	144	195	200	205	208
74	148	201	206	211	214
75	152	206	212	217	220
76	156	212	217	223	226
77	160	218	223	229	232
78	164	223	229	235	238
79	168	229	235	241	244
80	173	234	240	247	250

ARMY Female Height/Weight Chart

HEIGHT IN INCHES	MINIMUM WEIGHT	MAX WEIGHT AGE 17 - 20	MAX WEIGHT AGE 21 - 27	MAX WEIGHT AGE 28 - 39	MAX WEIGHT AGE 40 +
58	91	119	121	122	123
59	94	124	125	126	128
60	97	128	129	131	133
61	100	132	134	135	137
62	104	136	138	140	142
63	107	141	143	144	146
64	110	145	147	149	151
65	114	150	152	154	156
66	117	155	156	158	161
67	121	159	161	163	166
68	125	164	166	168	171
69	128	169	171	173	176
70	132	174	176	178	181
71	136	179	181	183	186
72	140	184	186	188	191
73	144	189	191	194	197
74	148	194	197	199	202
75	152	200	202	204	208
76	156	205	207	210	213
77	160	210	213	215	219
78	164	216	218	221	225
79	168	221	224	227	230
80	173	227	230	233	236

There are a few things that keep this table from being ideal. One is that the range is extremely wide. For example, at my height and age there is a 60 pound range from under weight to overweight. The next table is a little narrower. This is to compensate for the level of fitness. A more fit person is likely to be higher in the chart due to muscle mass.

MetLife height/weight table

This table is the most widely used, and most misunderstood. The table was created in 1943 from mortality statistics. Those living the longest tended to be in this height/weight range. It is not an endorsement of what is healthy, just what the longest-living people tend to be. On the other hand, this seems to be as reasonable a measure of healthy as anything – long life. Some criticisms of the table state that it did not take into consideration modern diets (that is to say the alarming trend toward obesity and the acceptance of it). Another criticism is that the table does not take into consideration the health and fitness addict of the modern age. In truth, this was developed in a time when people used their bodies more in day to day activities, walking, on the farm, bailing hay, etc., rather than finding fitness in the gym.   The end result, however, is probably very similar.

This table attempts to take into consideration body frame as a mitigating factor. Most of us assume that we know our frame size, or we select the large one because it allows us to have the most weight. The actual process for selecting frame size is described in the MetLife instructions as:

> "Bend forearm upward at a 90 degree angle. Keep fingers straight and turn the inside of your wrist toward your body. Place thumb and index finger of other hand on the two prominent bones on either side of the elbow. Measure space between your fingers on a ruler.(A physician would use a caliper.) Compare with tables below listing elbow measurements for **medium-framed** men and women. Measurements lower than those listed indicate small frame. Higher measurements indicate large frame."

ELBOW MEASUREMENTS FOR MEDIUM FRAME

Height in 1" heels **Men**	Elbow Breadth	Height in 1" heels **Women**	Elbow Breadth
5'2"-5'3"	$2_{1/2}$"-$2_{7/8}$"	4'10"-4'11"	$2_{1/4}$"-$2_{1/2}$"
5'4"-5'7"	$2_{5/8}$"-$2_{7/8}$"	5'0"-5'3"	$2_{1/4}$"-$2_{1/2}$"
5'8"-5'11"	$2_{3/4}$"-3"	5'4"-5'7"	$2_{3/8}$"-$2_{5/8}$"
6'0"-6'3"	$2_{3/4}$"-$3_{1/8}$"	5'8"-5'11"	$2_{3/8}$"-$2_{5/8}$"
6'4"	$2_{7/8}$"-$3_{1/4}$"	6'0"	$2_{1/2}$"-$2_{3/4}$"

Next, measure height in one-inch heels. The weight assumes 5 pounds of clothes for men and 3 pounds of clothes for women. One of the most accurate ways to compensate for this is to measure unclothed and add 5 for men and 3 for women.

For Men:

Height Feet Inches	Small Frame	Medium Frame	Large Frame
5' 2"	128-134	131-141	138-150
5' 3"	130-136	133-143	140-153
5" 4"	132-138	135-145	142-156
5' 5"	134-140	137-148	144-160
5' 6"	136-142	139-151	146-164
5' 7"	138-145	142-154	149-168
5' 8"	140-148	145-157	152-172
5' 9"	142-151	148-160	155-176
5' 10"	144-154	151-163	158-180
5' 11"	146-157	154-166	161-184
6' 0"	149-160	157-170	164-188
6' 1"	152-164	160-174	168-192
6' 2"	155-168	164-178	172-197
6' 3"	158-172	167-182	176-202
6' 4"	162-176	171-187	181-207

For Women:

Height Feet Inches	Small Frame	Medium Frame	Large Frame
4' 10"	102-111	109-121	118-131
4' 11"	103-113	111-123	120-134
5' 0"	104-115	113-126	122-137
5' 1"	106-118	115-129	125-140
5' 2"	108-121	118-132	128-143
5' 3"	111-124	121-135	131-147
5' 4"	114-127	124-138	134-151
5' 5"	117-130	127-141	137-155
5' 6"	120-133	130-144	140-159
5' 7"	123-136	133-147	143-163
5' 8"	126-139	136-150	146-167
5' 9"	129-142	139-153	149-170
5' 10"	132-145	142-156	152-173
5' 11"	135-148	145-159	155-176
6' 0"	138-151	148-162	158-179

Remember: Add 1 inch in height, and 3 pounds for women or 5 pounds for men. The frame size is selected by measuring the elbow and the chart represents the medium frame. Measurements above it are considered large framed and measurements below are small framed individuals.

Body fat percentage

This is becoming a more common way to measure what is considered healthy, although this method also has a few drawbacks. The most obvious is the difficulty in getting an accurate body fat percentage. Some scales provide a body fat percentage, but it fluctuates significantly depending on how much water you have in your system at the time of measurement.   There are several online calculators to help figure out the body fat percentage as well.

There is no absolute standard. Experts agree that some body fat is required, but finding that magic line between healthy and overweight varies somewhat. Women who enter the high end of athletic endeavors or the danger zone tend to stop menstruating, but that is the only objective indicator on what is too little body fat. Experts are all over the charts on what is acceptable. The chart below is simply a place to start; again, the best measure is between you and your mirror, and what you are comfortable with. You will notice that some of the percentages overlap when it comes to the "Performance Athlete" category. This is because the lower end of the standard Healthy category can also be in the Athlete category.   The most widely used percentages are:

Male Age	Dangerous	Performance Athlete	Healthy	Overweight	Obese
17-40	< 5%	6 – 13%	8-19%	19 – 25%	Over 25%
41-60	< 6%	7 – 15%	11 - 22%	22 – 27%	Over 27%
60 - 80	< 5%	7 – 15%	13 - 25%	25 – 30%	Over 30%

Female Age	Dangerous	Performance Athlete	Healthy	Overweight	Obese
17-40	< 14%	14 - 20%	21-33%	33-39%	Over 39%
41-60	< 15%	15 - 22%	23 -35%	35-40%	Over 40%
61 - 80	< 15%	15 - 23%	24 – 36%	36-42%	Over 42%

Before and After

The pictures in this section are of real people, ones just like you who did this program at home, using the plan as outlined in this book. The before and after pictures are of the same people, not two separate actors, or retouched to create an illusion; they are as honest as we can make them. Because the program is meant to be done at home, the pictures are taken by the individuals in their homes. Uniformly, those who did not take pictures regretted the lack of comparison at the end of the program or round. Take pictures; you don't have to share them, but if you want to, you will never have the opportunity to take them again. The pictures are also excellent motivators when you can see the scale move, but you are not sure that there is progress. The pictures don't always show you the perfectly fit body at the end, not everyone is there yet…but they are on the way. We have selected a variety of progress shots and a variety of body types and ages to show the differences. The very large and the only slightly overweight people find equal effectiveness in the program. A variety of body types are shown, as well as loss stages depicted. I'm thrilled that some of my friends have allowed me to share their stories with you., Let me introduce you to my Amazing Shrinking Friends.

Let's start with Me

There is nothing worse than a diet book that is written by someone who has never been overweight, they don't *know*, they don't understand. It is something you know when you walk in those shoes. I was motivated to find an answer because I was relentlessly putting on a half pound to a full pound a month, every month, and I just couldn't make it stop no matter how much exercise or healthy eating I did. I went to doctor after doctor and they told me it was not an issue, or not to worry about it. Some humored me and referred me to nutritionists. Nothing worked until I found this program, and translated it into something that could be done at home by everyone. I had my doubts, but figured I did not have anything to lose. I felt fantastic while working on the program and thrilled to be able to share it with my friends. Every pound they lost was a victory for me as well. My problems came mostly from my clothes falling off me, and needing to update my wardrobe faster than I could bring myself to get rid of old clothes. My fashion sense - which has never been stellar to begin with - needed a complete overhaul because nothing in the closet fit. I took to buying the same style of jeans and measuring myself by how long it took me to fit into the next lower size. The largest surprise for me was that my shape changed. I had always been a 'pear' shape, and heavy in the legs and butt. I realized that even at my best weight before, I was a different shape and I probably had a different ideal weight. I've never been below a 12 before, now I am wearing a 4. I lost 61 pounds.

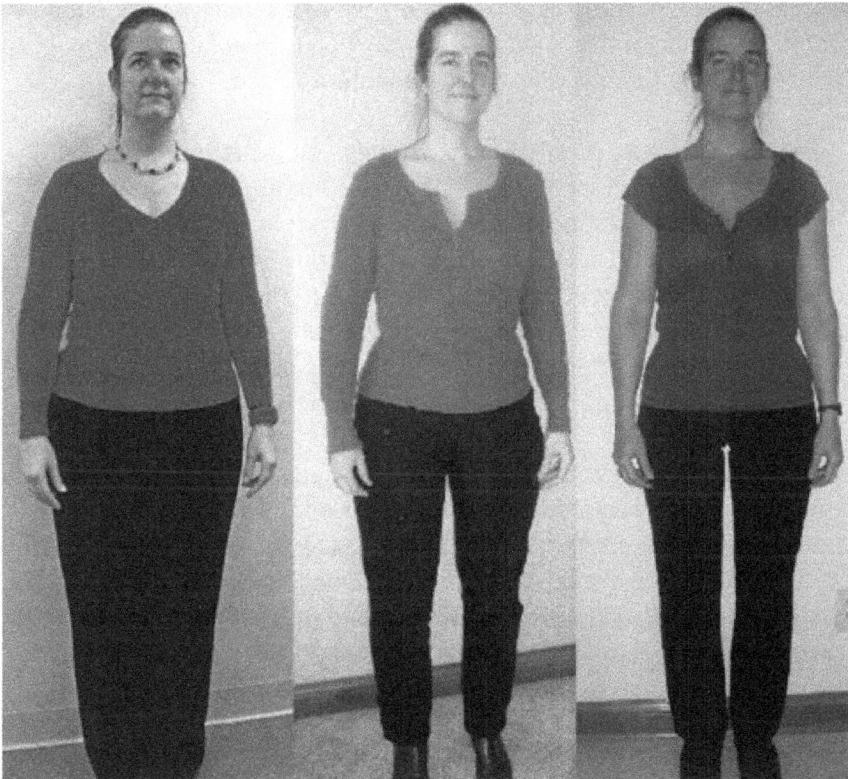

My pictures – Before, Round 1, and another half round

Angie and Brian

Angie is a late-thirties mother of four. Like many she has an active life (she has four children!) and tries to take care of herself. She hates that her body shape makes her look perpetually pregnant, and it is a constant source of embarrassment to constantly be asked when she is due, or queried on if she has enough children already.

It's not like she has a sedentary life, or does not look after her health. A year before starting this program she finished a 90-day extreme workout cycle and loved how it gave her muscles, but was infuriated that at the end of the program her stomach was actually LARGER than before. Her doctor informed her that she had a great layer of muscle, right under the fat...and she still had a large stomach.

Angie had one more problem...she had been on heart and blood pressure medication for 12 years. She talked to her doctor about the program and was cautioned that she should not lose more than 10% of her body weight before coming in and getting her medication adjusted at their next appointment in 30 days. The Doctor did not seem to be delivering that requirement with any kind of conviction, because people just don't lose that much in 30 days. Well, Angie and her husband went into the program and followed it exactly.

Within a week, they had little to no appetite and found that the meals they thought they wanted they could not even finish. The most popular vegetable for them was spinach - fresh, steamed, rolled around chicken, in a soup, you name it. They drank about a gallon of water a day each, and were full and satisfied most of the time. The occasional gathering of friends was a challenge, but they packed their own food, and used flavored water to satisfy the taste for something different.

Angie's husband started taking in his uniform pants, and found his shirts fit looser almost immediately. Angie was not so sure, because she had been wearing drawstring pants and elastic waists for so long, it was not as obvious. At three weeks, disaster happened; Angie's husband was taken to the doctor for severe kidney stones. They were worried that the diet had caused them, or made the problem worse. The urologist explained that the stones he had were very large, and had been developing for years. The diet (high in spinach and water) is what probably broke them up and washed them out of his system before they required surgery. That alone was incentive to finish up the program, and at four weeks, her husband had lost the maximum weight.

At five weeks, Angie started to feel light headed, and needed a nap during the day. She held out until her next doctor's appointment, but really felt run down and exhausted. When she went to the Doctor, she found that her blood pressure was drastically too low, and she realized she had failed to follow the warning from the doctor about losing more than 10% of her weight...even the doctor had not said it with much conviction. Angie had just lost 28 pounds in a little over a month.

Needless to say, this kind of drastic sudden weight loss can be cause for alarm, particularly in the eyes of doctors who regularly tell their patients to lose weight only to see them struggle without success time and again. No matter how much gushing Angie did about how fantastic she felt on the plan, or how much she and her husband lost, the doctor was concerned that Angie had developed an eating disorder. They made a deal. If Angie's weight stayed the same for 30 days, the doctor would consider her to be someone who beat the odds and lost the weight, and reduced her blood pressure. But if she lost more, she would go to a psychiatric consultation. In the meantime, Angie's doctor had her stop taking her blood pressure medication, severely reduce the heart medication and take only one pill for water. Fortunately, the next 30 days was also in the plan as the 'maintenance' phase of the program, where the objective is to keep the weight exactly where it is.

Angie came back in 30 days, whereupon her doctor removed her from all of her blood pressure medication, heart medication and water pills, for the first time in 12 years.

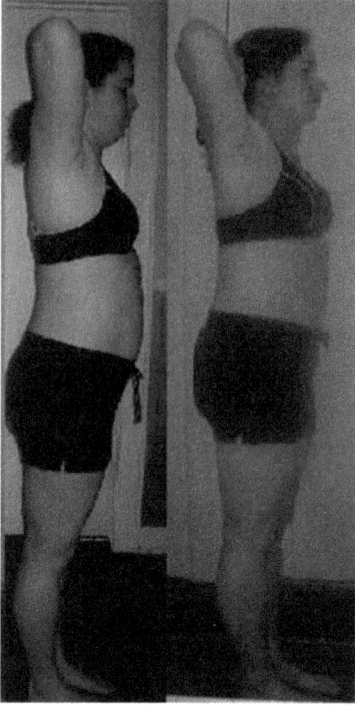

Angie – .5 rounds   Angie – 1.5 rounds

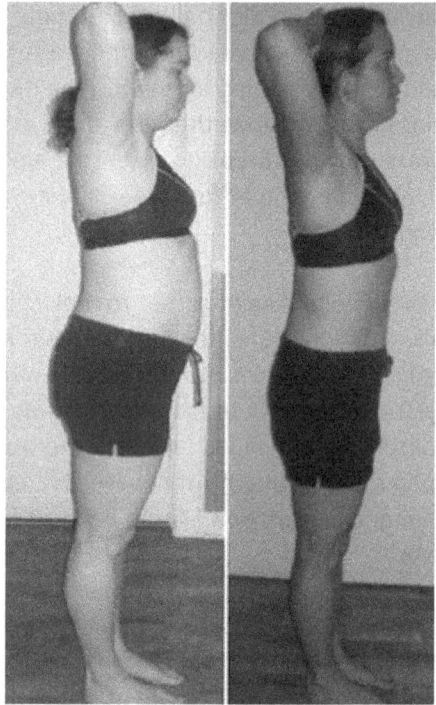

Nancy F

Nancy is a pessimist turned evangelist. She started by watching her friend dramatically lose weight, and wanted to try. She is an early fifty-something who has had a hard life. Several car accidents have left her in pain and hardly able to move without medication. She also has a zest for life and all of its flavors, and enjoys being active and engaged. Her will and her body collide regularly and reach a truce through significant medication and pain management. The average day had her taking the maximum allowable dose of morphine, as well as other pain management medication.

While she was reading the program, she was sure it was too good to be true. She had tried low calorie diets before and was always hungry. She had tried exercise programs that she could not even bear the thought of now, due to the constant pain she suffered. She was sure that this would not work, and she was practically going through withdrawals at the very thought of giving up her beloved diet cola. Nancy was also sure that she could lose 40 pounds in a round, and be fine, she would just tough it out until she did. She was disappointed to be told that she was allowed no more than 34 pounds......just a few more won't make a difference, right? No, it does make a difference. The idea is to permanently remove the weight. Taking off too much without giving the body a chance to adjust is just as bad as cheating throughout the program.

She was sure she would lose it from her chest, the one place she did not want to lose. She was sure she would be hungry. She was sure she would have no energy. She was sure that in a few weeks, she would be right where she was before...and that is what gave her the impetus to try. In a few weeks, she would either have no change, or dramatic change...she had nothing to lose (except the weight).

In about a week she found that she all but had to force herself to eat, she just was not interested in the food she was allowed, or any food for that matter. It is important to note that if you have no appetite, it is vital to have at least the protein in order to keep your body from finding protein in your muscles and going after them. She stuck with it, ate what she could, and found she started losing rapidly.

A couple of weeks into the program she had the opportunity to work on the pond she had always wanted to build in her backyard. Her energy was up, and she went out to move rocks. Normally the exercise would have destroyed her - not because she did not have the muscle, but because her damaged frame and nerves would have screamed at the abuse. The next morning she got up and worked on the project some more, only to realize that she had not needed her pain killers. In fact, she did not feel all that sore at all and marveled at the thought that she could move more freely, and without pain, than she could in recent memory.

Nancy capped out at the maximum 34 pounds in the first round, and found a few surprising things. She thought she could strive for 40 pounds tops, and when she lost 34 she found her shape had changed significantly. She no longer carried her weight around the middle, and her body was developing a noticeable figure. She realized she could lose more, and now knew how to do so effortlessly to have one of those fashion-ready bodies she thought she would never see again. She is now down 53 pounds, and is looking forward to seeing what else comes off. The program will not dip into Normal or Structural fat, so all she has to lose is the Abnormal fat.

Shopping has become a challenge for her; she tries on clothes she thinks are the correct size only to have them fall off her. It seems to be a common problem with the group, size changes so quickly that it is hard to keep up a good mental picture of what we look like.

After completing a full round and stabilizing for a couple of weeks, Nancy went to her regular doctor for a check-up and a refill on her medication. The doctor's jaw hit the floor. He said she was ten years younger in vitality, stature and overall look. I have to agree, so does Nancy. The doctor is now exploring the program for his patients.

Mr. and Mrs. H (Steve and Nancy)

Mr. H was mostly concerned for his wife, and was willing to do the program to support her in her efforts. Great guy. He figured he could lose a little, and that would not hurt, but his primary motivation was to provide her support. When he looked at his before pictures however, he was appalled. He knew he could lose some, but did not realize how much.

They joined the program, started up and started losing right away. While they were happy losing 4 and 5 pounds in the first week, such a loss was worth examining. Normally, the loss in the first couple of weeks is more dramatic. We looked at exactly what they were eating and found a few hidden cheats they never intended to take. Imitation crab had been a staple for a fresh summer salad; unfortunately, there are all sorts of items in that package that are not on the list. Chemicals, hidden starches, coloring, and all manner of other items that our eyes just glance over when reading the ingredient list were in clear evidence, and had slowed them down.

They began to read packages more carefully, if it is in the package, and not on the list, it is not in the plan. This simple rule goes for anything that claims to be 'no calorie' or 'healthy' or anything else. Not on the list – not on the plan. It is heartbreaking to see people come so close

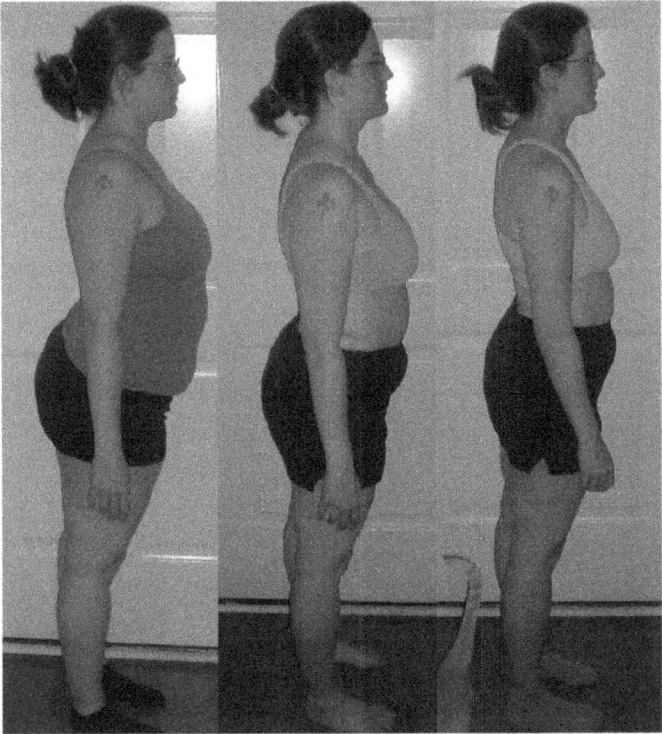

Nancy H after two rounds

to sticking to the plan, only to have the unintentional cheat creep up on them and prevent them from getting the most out of it.

They came to the conclusion that fresh meals were the only way to go, in order to be sure, and sure enough, the weight started dropping even faster. Mrs. H lost 25 and Mr. H lost 30 in the first round. They are now up to 50 for her and 40 for him.

Once finished, and looking at his pictures, Mr. H can't wait to start the next round, he is finding a V cut to his body he had not expected, and Mrs. H was thrilled to find that her jeans zipped up without her having to lie down to zip them. Most surprising to her was the belly that she had from carrying two children began to recede. That alone made it worth doing again! In addition, they noticed that their posture changed. They stood up straighter, could look people in the eye better, rather than looking up from a head bent over, they were less

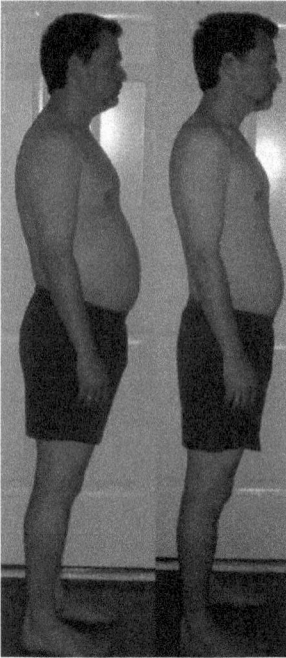

tired at the end of the day because they were not fighting their bodies just to walk and stand. Mr. H realized he was being taken more seriously at work – fit and healthy people are perceived as better leaders, and it was showing.

Their pictures show them at the completion of the first round, and they can't wait to go again! The largest change for him was in the stomach, for her, in the rear. They both noticed a change in the neck and overall right away.

Steve after 1 Round

Liz

Liz wanted to lose 20 pounds. I would have told you that she did not have that much to lose at all, but she insisted, and pointed out that her proportions were not what they should be, particularly for her family. This is a program about personal choice, and it will not let you lose anything but the Abnormal fat, so she gave it a try.

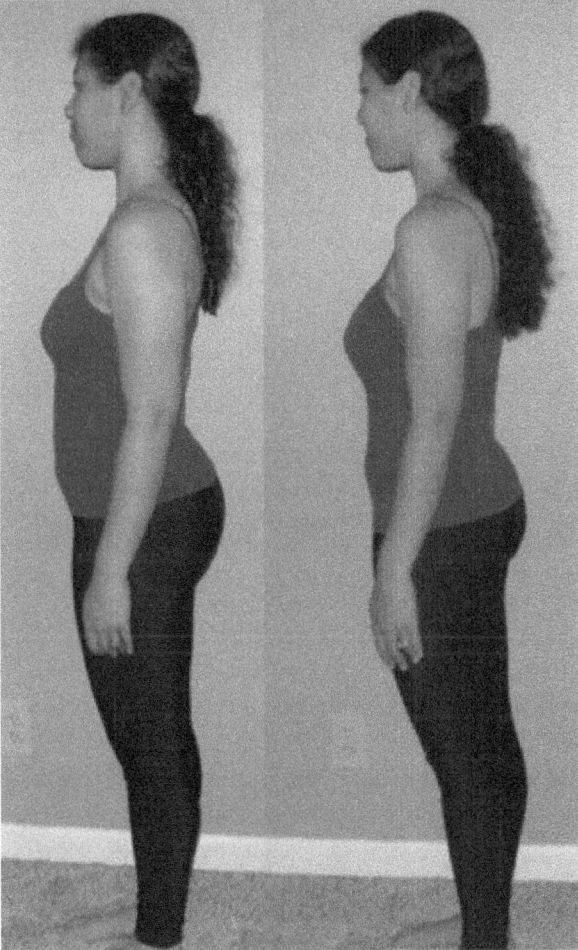

At four weeks, she had what she wanted. Twenty pounds down, no exercise to do it, a vibrant healthy outlook and a huge smile. Losing the weight also changed her posture. She lost in the rear, stomach and chin, and the overall layer of excess that she had always disliked.

Liz after 4 weeks

Tim

Tim saw me just after I had completed the second round, and he had not seen me for months…..his jaw hit the floor, and he asked how, I told him, and we got to work. He dove right in and read the plan, agreed to stick to it, made his order and began. Unfortunately, he did not have a scale, but used the very accurate one at work, and gave himself a weekly weigh in on Monday morning.

The first week he realized he was not all that hungry, but some things just look good. There is a process to go through where the brain sorts out the difference between what it wants and what it needs. He did not need that wedding cake the first weekend, but boy he wanted it! Many of us believe we know the difference, and we may even have a good handle on it. The truth is, you can never distinguish the difference between need and want until one of them is completely gone. On this program, need is gone, all that is left is want. It is an eye-opening experience for most people.

Tim experienced a heart breaking stall for nearly a week; it was frustrating and demotivating, and just plain depressing. Here he was going along losing 12 pounds in the first week only to have that stall.

Rather than give up, he stuck it out, and upped his water intake to a gallon a day. His body was busy rearranging and dissolving fat. To do this, the body needed to hang onto a little extra water for a short time. A few days later, he was losing a pound or three a day, and was back on track fairly quickly. He lost his maximum of 34 pounds with three days to spare, and even though his first pictures are taken with a shirt on, you can still see that the shirt fits looser, and he has shrunk a little all over, particularly under the chin. He is getting married soon, and his largest concern is going to be getting the right fit on the tux!

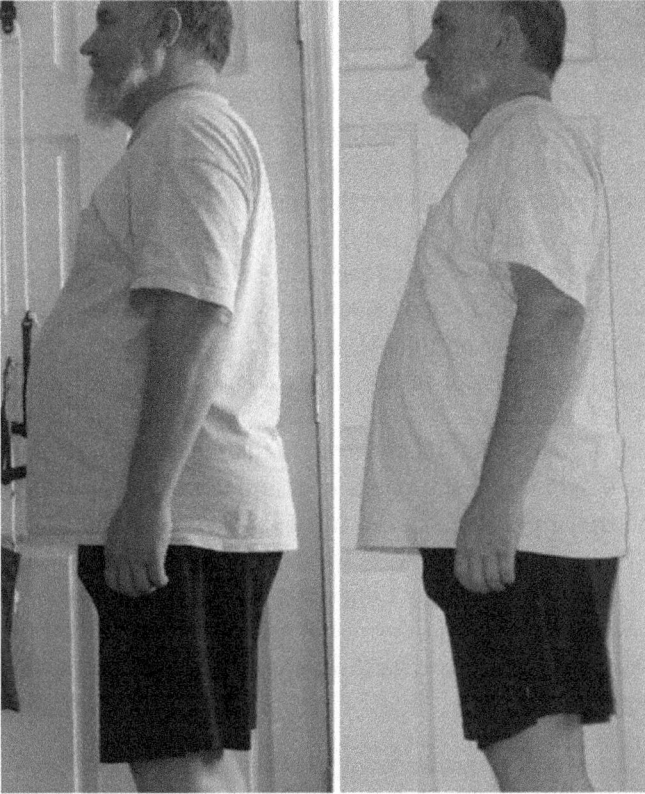

Tim after 1 Round

Kathy

Kathy saw me after the first round and sat me down and demanded I spill my guts…..no problem. We talked about how to get her started and she set out on her plan. She tried to enlist the camaraderie of friends to do the program with her, and was shocked at what she heard.   She could point to me and say she knew it worked, there was living proof…but they wouldn't join her. Mostly they just said, diet and exercise are fine for me. What can you do? Diet and exercise are fine, but they have limits, and asking a very heavy person to apply the same diet and exercise program that a svelte person does is not reasonable and just plain harder than it has to be.

For her, the most dramatic change occurred in the stomach and neck. But she also lost weight in the shoulders, rear and hips. In a couple of days she noticed the appetite had gone away, and she began to examine the differences between need and want, and discovered that she wanted, but did not need many things. Her sweet tooth was satisfied with SweetLeaf™ in liquid form that she could add to water, and generally found that she could go through her day without making great modifications.

Again, her shape had changed. She had stored her weight in the mid section and she was now developing an hourglass figure. No more did she have the matronly figure of a mother of two…now it was more a matter of the flattering figure of a healthy, active, vibrant woman. Her largest loss in the first round was to her stomach and rear, and of course the chin. Somewhat surprisingly, her back also lost a great deal, and her posture improved.   Her second round was a half round as she caught a bad cold and had to take cough medicine with lots of sugar, so that round was short; however, there was still a dramatic difference. Her pictures have a wind chime in the background, and this made it easier to line up the pictures, but it also showed a dramatic improvement in her posture…look at the angle of her glasses over time, her head is not being forced down by the fat in her neck, and it is more natural for her to look up, and stand up.

Kathy also complained, sort of, about having to get new bras. Not because the cup size changed, but because the body size changed! Her husband is not at all upset with this development.

Those friends? At the end of her second round, Kathy was down over 40 pounds. Her friends had not changed their weight at all, except for the ones that gained.

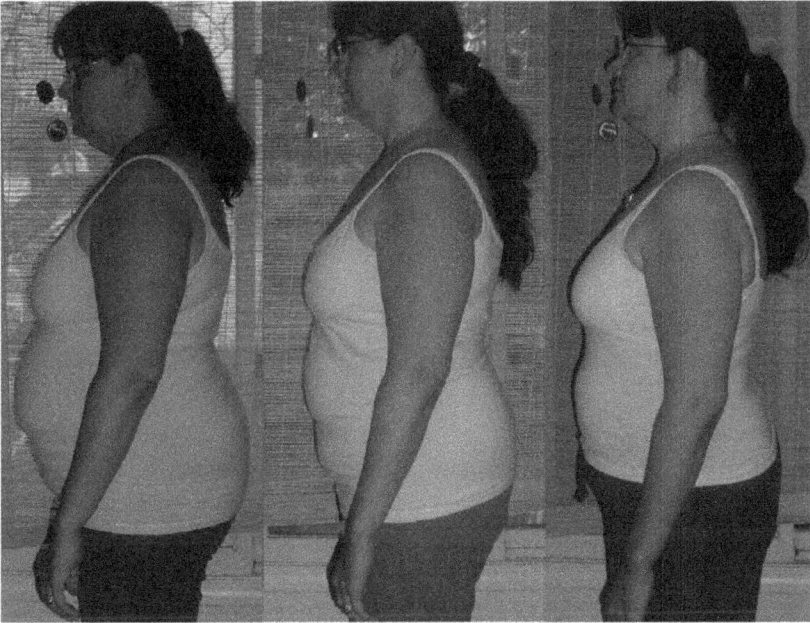

Kathy – Before, Round 1 and 1.5 Rounds

"B"

B is a friend from work. We had commiserated together a number of times that weight just should not be this hard to lose. As a 5' 4" blond German woman, she has the typical heavy German round body. When she came to the US she was thin, athletic and...well...svelte. Year after year she saw herself gain weight, so she went on a diet, lost a little, and gained it back, then gained more. She would eat a lunch that would make a rabbit hungry, and still she lost nothing. She was thrilled to be able to lose a pound or two by walking a couple of miles a day at work, but even that did not last.

After a while, she was still very round, and it was painful to walk more than a few yards as her feet and knees were constantly sore. Her body was consuming Structural fat in order to compensate for the reduced calories, and had robbed her of the cushion on the bottom of her feet. It was heartrending to see her suffer, but what could she do, 'diet and exercise' was all she heard from her doctor. She went to holistic medical practitioners when modern medicine failed her, she tried acupuncture, acupressure, hypnotism, protein- and fat-based diets, diet food plans, you name it; in the two years I worked with her, she was always trying something new. And none of it worked.

B is very observant and was the first person to say anything to me. I was three weeks into the diet, 15 sudden pounds down, and she was the first person to actually ask. She researched it herself and found what I found. I showed her the pros and cons of everyone's opinions out there and she plunged right in, realizing that she could not feel worse than she currently did.

She experienced an odd phenomena that a few people independently reported: phantom emotions. B put on much of her weight while going through a violent, dangerous separation from an abusive person. She lived a portion of her life in true fear of her life. As she lost the weight, she found that some shadow of that emotion was stored chemically in the fat. There would be days that she suddenly felt momentarily apprehensive for no reason at all. By the time she could identify the emotion, it was gone, but she recognized it as the flavor of the emotion she felt when she had put on the weight to begin with. A couple of people have expressed a similar reaction, and are all too happy to have that chemical trash removed.

After the first round she lost what she called her 'back boobs.' But a larger change took place between her ears. For the first time she could eat without regret or guilt. If she put on weight, so what, she knew how to take it off now without significant effort. In fact, as a test to herself she *tried* to put weight on between rounds. She went out of her way to snack and have fattening fast food frozen concoctions and she did manage to put on a couple of pounds...and promptly lost them again a few days later. For her the largest change came in her relationship with food. It was pleasurable, without guilt, enjoyable without regret, flavorful without the need to gorge. This program does not teach you how to look at food differently; it changes your taste and views if you let it.

B will be doing additional rounds, and now knows she can take off the weight at whatever pace she wants. She is in control of her body for the first time in her adult life and couldn't be happier about it.

Amy

I bleed for Amy. She is a young, vibrant wonderful person who has always been the 'chubby' girl. Not so much fat, but always has the round face and extra padding. She too had been on every diet known to man, and was willing to try anything to get rid of those pounds.

Unfortunately, she had the one thing that will undermine the program every time, a deliberate saboteur. Her husband did not want her to 'lose the junk in your trunk,' as he would tell her. And while she would try to stick to the plan, he would offer up every enticement possible to derail her. Take her to dinner, bring in her favorite take-out or delivery, and bring home sweets and cakes. It took her a while to realize that there were more of these behaviors while she was on the program than before she started, and realize it was his way of making sure she did not lose weight.

The interesting thing is, he is much larger than she. It does not take a rocket scientist to guess there is a concern not for her losing weight, but for him. Even so, she lost more than a dozen pounds in the six weeks and kept it off. I bleed for her because she put so much effort into the program, only to be stripped from the full effect.

There is an important lesson here, though. Some people do not want to lose weight; they see it as part of their personality, or identity. Some have used their substantial size as the catch all reason for people not accepting them, and if they lose the weight, they may have to take a hard look at their personal behavior if they still feel unaccepted, and that can be both scary and intimidating. Make sure you want to lose weight, because it will happen this time, and happen quickly.

Crystal

Crystal is funny, young and sure of herself. I told her the program was exacting, not hard, but exacting. She took a little cheat here or there, and was sure it would not make a difference. The entire team pointed out to her that time is a limiting factor; you have 42 days to lose weight, no more. After those 42 days you must stop because the body becomes immune to the HCG and the last thing you want to do is build up that immunity.

She is young, and 42 days is a long time...until you reach the end of it.

She had a little left in her bottle and wanted to continue so she could lose just a few more pounds. There had been weeks where she did not lose any weight because she had cheated a little here and there, but she was not worried about it at the time. Until time ran out. No, that's all in a round, 42 days, no more. Then a six week wait.

Usually, during that six weeks people are very anxious to start again. They want to lose more, but realize they have to stop, or risk not losing any more on the program. It is a tough restriction to impose on oneself, but necessary. The upshot is that she understands the value of time as she started her second round, and was the model of plan adherence. She stalled a few times, but understood that this was normal as the body moves through weights that it maintained for a long time in the past. She has completed the second round, and is down 40 pounds…..she may well take off more, and now knows she can at any time. (Update in second edition: She did lose more, and quickly…..the next round she stayed on the plan.)

Susan

Susan was another co-worker, and a scientist. She saw the results in me, and wanted to try. She did her research, as I encourage everyone to do, and she found multiple articles on the perils of the program. And like I did, she looked closer. The articles she found were largely by two people, and they simply referenced each other's articles……..kind of like a circular argument. The 'studies' had no specifics, and no publication in medical journals. The cautions were against ultra low calorie diets, but not ones supplemented by HCG. There were those that decried the value of homeopathic HCG

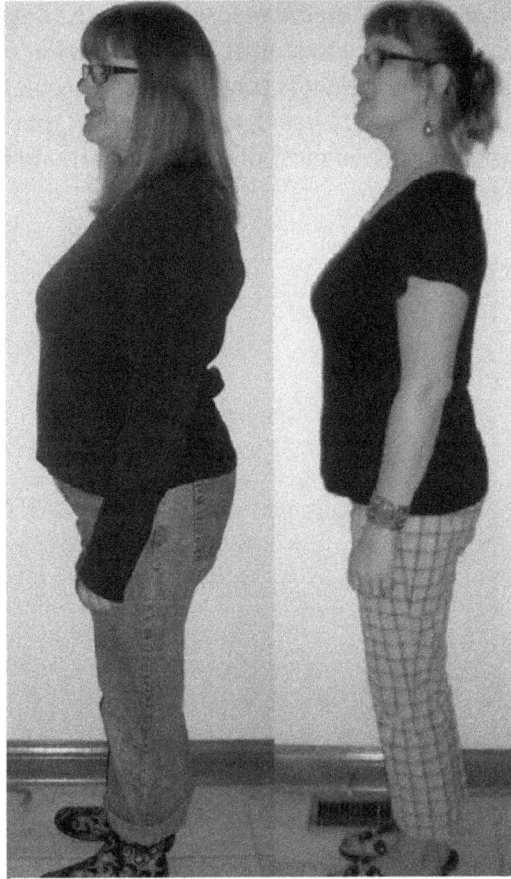

Susan after 1.5 rounds

and by extension all HCG, but none that actually addressed the original protocol as given by the original clinic. Susan jumped in.

As with many people on the program, she did not really see the difference in herself. Yes, of course she could see the scale move every day, but that is still hard to see on the body when you see yourself every morning and night. Her husband noticed though. He could tell her, but she could discount that to him being supportive. It was not until she put her pants on one day and they fell off that she realized he might not just be offering idle flattery.

She was sure she would not see her skin shrink up after three kids, but while she was on the second round, she began to see just that. She is not sure where to stop at this point, as her shape is changing as she is losing. The weight is coming off the 'problem areas' first. I've known her for nearly 10 years, and she admits that I've never seen her this size before, and most of the people around her can't even remember her at this size.

Reed

Reed is a healthy man in his late 40's who has a desk job that has allowed him to develop a standard middle age 'spread'. Like most people, it crept up on him in little stages and was common enough not to be overly embarrassing. Somewhere in there, there had to be a little embarrassment, because when he started the program no one could get him to take the "Before" pictures. Fortunately, his wife had pictures from their vacation in Hawaii. He started the program at an all-time high for him of 258, and ended at 195 two and a half rounds later, a weight he has not seen since high school.

His largest challenge was realizing that even though he felt great he had to curb his exercise; doing too much is exhausting and counterproductive to the program. He is not a fan of diets, and not really the kind of guy you would expect to stick to any kind of diet, but he found the program easy. Clothes that were difficult or too tight to wear were comfortable again, and every day he is stunned at the results and surprised at how straightforward and predictable the plan is.

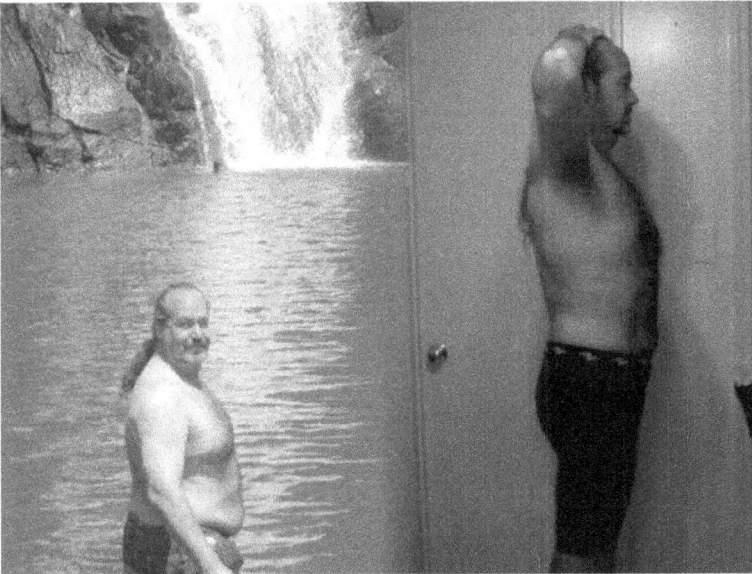

Reed after two rounds

Kim

I've known Kim for years, and we have both struggled with diets together. We've tried encouraging each other and helping where we could, but like most, we experienced the same hopes and heartaches that most dieters have when something works for awhile, and stops. Kim worked with me at a distance and like many, had lots of questions, and did lots of research.

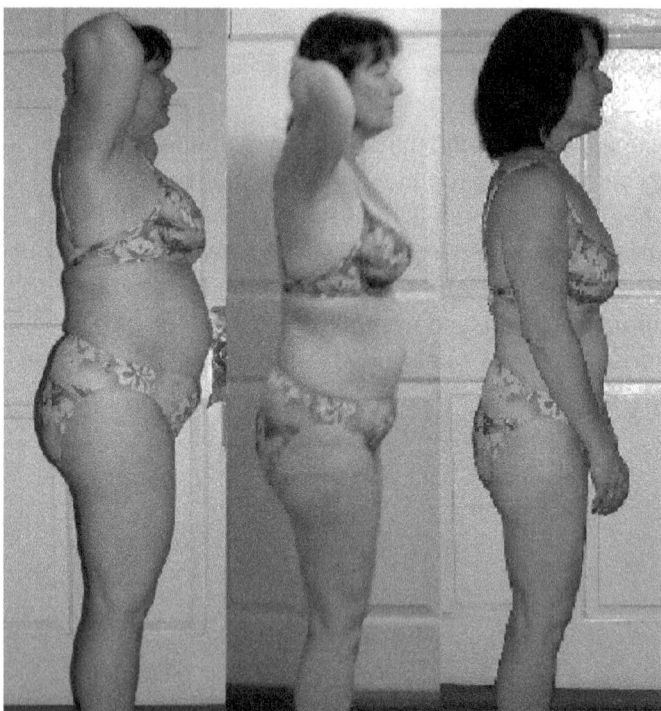

Kim after two rounds

For her, the program worked flawlessly, though she had hoped she would lose more than 20 pounds the first round. For her, she did the program perfectly, but still did not lose more than 20......stop......try to say this with a straight face......."I only lost 20 pounds in six weeks......" It's amazing how our perception of success changes. When you hear yourself saying "I only lost 5 pounds this week," slap yourself for me, and laugh.

In her case, the body spent quite a bit of time reorganizing rather than actively losing. The next round, however, continued to take off more weight, and every time her overall shape develops into a more proportioned body. This is something she has never experienced in her adult life, and is getting the body back she had in high school.

Update for the second edition: The last picture of Kim was taken only a few months ago. She wanted to show that not only had she lost the weight, but it had stayed off. Although it is hard to tell in these pictures, the bikini top is tied in place as it was 'indecent' not to.

Cameron

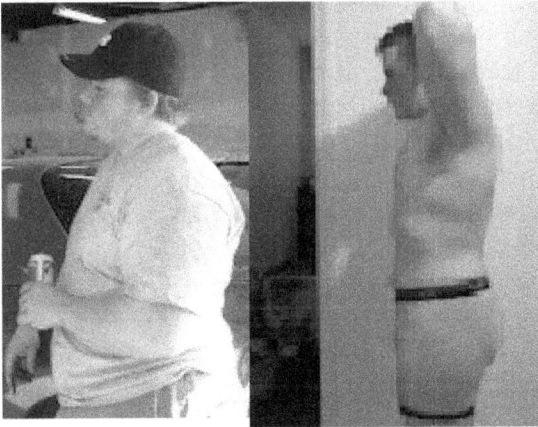

Cameron after two rounds

Cameron was getting ready to go into the military. He was a bit overweight. OK, he was a lot overweight. In fact he had struggled with his weight all his life, but college made it difficult to keep in check. He knew that he would not be able to get through Basic Training down at the Benning Home for Boys (Army Infantry School) if he did not take off the weight first. He set about the program with his usual diligence and actively attacked the problem. Some of those close to him tried to tease him out of it, like his father who cooked eggs and waved them under his nose. He took the plate and tossed Dad's eggs in the trash, and went back to eating his apple. Or the time his girlfriend teased him with a fresh bag of potato chips that he took and crunched up into pieces, before handing them back to her. Cameron can be single minded when he chooses to be. He lost the full 32 pounds in 21 days, and then did a second round and maxed out at 23 days. With a total loss of over 65 pounds, he went to Ft. Benning and did fine in the Summer Georgia heat.

Kathy HT

Kathy, as my realtor, was one of the first people to welcome me to my new state, and help me find a house. She is also an active grandmother and running her own business. She is the picture of active. But she has also been carrying around a few extra pounds. She saw the success other team members were having, and signed on. She has completed two rounds and went on a cruise and kept the weight off. She was down 40 pounds and plans to continue. She was one of our oldest team members, but clearly indicated that it worked as well, if not better, on her than the younger members. I attribute the difference to her willingness to stick to the plan faithfully. *Second edition update:* She lost a total of 60 pounds, kept it off for two years and is incredibly happy with the results. People constantly stop her and ask her how and what she did. What I like about the last picture is her posture. Look at the angle of her glasses. It was not staged, but it shows how much the person changes. She said one of her biggest surprises was having her Doctor tell her that she was at a healthy weight, and that she did not need to lose any more! First time she had walked away from the Dr. Office with perfect blood pressure, heart rate and weight – and a guilt free, healthy smile on her face.

Kathy has kept it off for over two years now, and could not be happier.

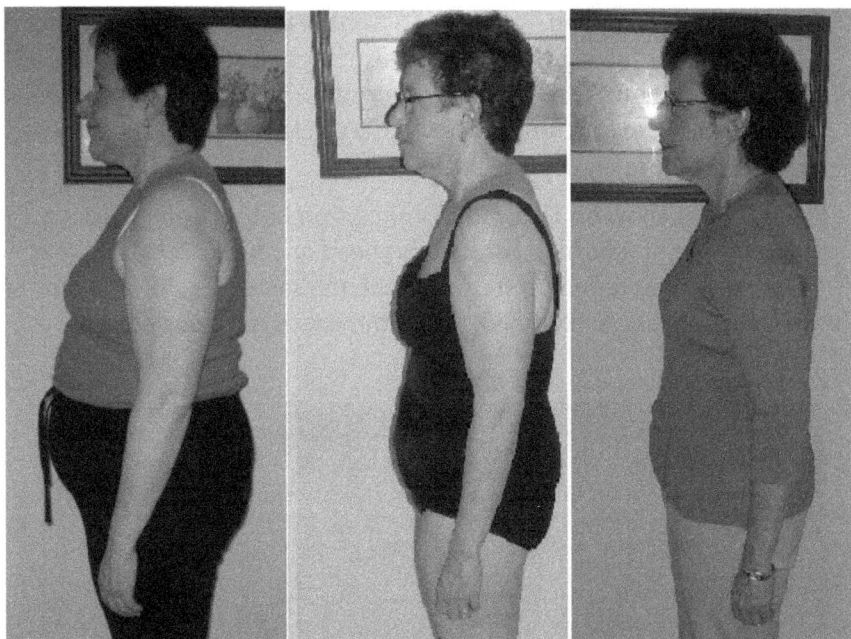

Kathy – Before, During and After 3 rounds

Tina and Rob V

Tina is another friend from work. She (in my opinion) could not possibly have a weight problem, but she felt she did. And that really is the stunning thing, our own perceptions are what count here. She was worried, asked a million questions and was one of the most insistent that we get a hard copy of this book created so that she could hand it to people.

Once she started her fears about drinking enough went away. Her concerns about being hungry went away. Her worry that they would not have enough variety went away. Her worry that she could not fit it into her active life style dissolved.

Her husband was already plotting ways to get around the strict structure of the program, but Tina was insistent and they went at it together.

Tina lost a full 20 pounds, all that she wanted to, and happily started shopping in her teenage daughter's closet. Rob lost 34 pounds and has also kept it off. They now kick themselves for not taking before and after pictures, but Tina did have two similar pictures taken a year apart, one before and one after the diet.

While it does show on Tina, it really shows on Rob as well, there is a dramatic loss of 'thickness' around his head and neck. Tina's 17 year old protests that her mom should not be the same size she is……but with more shape. Sorry, child, that is the way it is suppose to be.

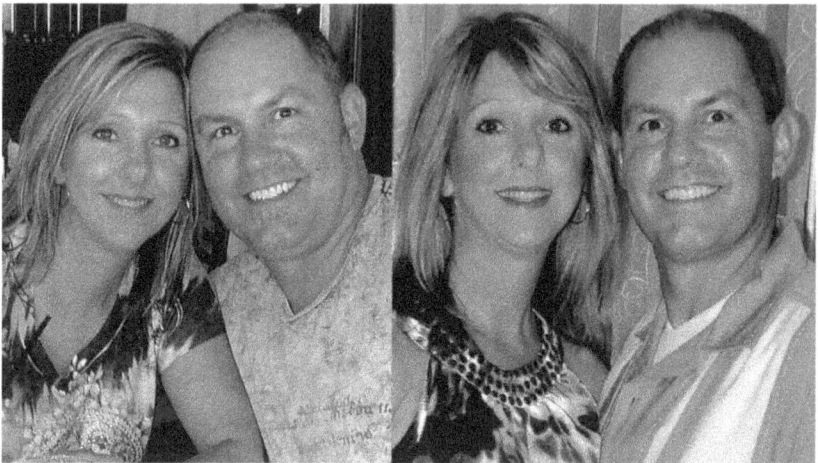

Rob and Tina – One round

Dale N

Never assume you are too large to start this program. Dale started at over 400 lbs, and has already lost 100 in the last year. He has taken time off now and then to do travel or for special activities, but he is well on his way to losing the weight for life. He moves better, feels better and is making a huge difference in his life and outlook. He is one of my favorites to keep an eye on, because I only see him occasionally, and every time I do, there is less of him, and I know he is getting the body he has always wanted and could not have before. He is a true inspiration. I hope to be able to have pictures of him by the time we publish again.

Your Pictures

All of the pictures above are people just like you. They tried diets, could not lose weight, or gained weight after. They struggled to control weight, sometimes their entire life. With this program they found a fix, a long term solution to weight gain. Every person who faithfully did the program lost twenty pounds or more the first round. Every person. Male, female, young adult, middle aged or older...every person. After the program they ate what they wanted to eat, and kept it off.

Take pictures. Start now even. Take a picture of yourself today; you don't have to share it. But, honestly, those who didn't wished they HAD so they had the comparison to see or show off!

Tips for taking great pictures:

- Stand in front of a reference point, like a door or wall with markings that won't move (this will help size the picture for comparison, as people tend to gain height and loose all over size),
- Take the same pose each time
- Take a front, back and side view,
- Wear close fitting clothes, and the same clothes if you can, or similar clothes if you are falling out of the ones you started with.

They don't have to be professional quality, they don't have to be taken by someone else if you can figure out how to set the timer on the camera, just take them. When you do this program you will never be this size again, and you will lose the opportunity to have this comparison and be able to inspire others.

If you decide not to do this program that's ok, put a date on your calendar to take another picture six weeks from now. Compare the two pictures at the end of six weeks, and ask yourself if they are similar to the results above. If they are not, consider doing this program. If you want help getting started, staying on the program or asking questions, drop me a note at Tobi@fat2fab.org and I'll link you to a Facebook page where you can talk to others on the program. You can leave any time you want, or stay to share and encourage others. The team is a great place to ask questions and here first hand advice and tips. We keep it a private group so the people there are willing to share details.

Because the program is not that difficult, it really is hard to 'see' the results until you compare them at the end. Don't get me wrong, they are there, really, it is just hard to believe that it is happening. Most people don't realize how much they have changed without the pictures.

If you take pictures, and you are willing to show, send them to us! We would love to see your progress, and hear your story! You can send them to mystory@fat2fab.org. If you let us, we may even publish your story and pictures, but we won't do that, of course, unless you are willing to share. If you don't want to share, that's ok too. It is a deeply personal thing, and believe me, I understand, I've been there. I've felt the frustration, the let down, the hopelessness of feeling like I had to accept being overweight. However, I have felt the success and elation at completing this program and moving from fat to fab! So take the pictures. If you change your mind (and most do when they see the results) it is the only way to see the full impact. I hope you will become one of my Amazing Shrinking Friends, and I look forward to hearing from you.

The Cookbook!

There are many HCG diet recipes on the web, unfortunately many of them are 'low cal' but include items that are not on the list.......don't use these. Zucchini, broccoli, cauliflower, oranges and olive oil are not on the list, and I can't tell you how many "HCG recipes" I've seen that include them. They may be considered "healthy", but for this program, they are not acceptable.

The following pages have over 100 recipes with variations that substitute one type of meat for another. Every recipe in here sticks to the protocol EXACTLY. There are spice combinations, soups, vegetables, whole entrees and desserts. There are more than enough to have a new recipe for every meal on a full six week cycle.

Remember; don't have the same meal twice in a row. Make sure that if an entrée uses a vegetable, you don't also make another vegetable dish in that meal. That is to say, one protein, one vegetable, one fruit in each meal. Make sure not to overload the amount of a vegetable used. Use the chart in the Phase 2 section of the book to measure an 'allowable amount' of a vegetable to make sure you don't go over 500 calories in a day.

These recipes come from all over, some from the experimentation of team members, others from various web sites and books and adjusted to stay within the program. An excellent place online for additional recipes is HCGrecipes.blogspot.com. They have a great track record of sticking to the program in their recipes. Sparkpeople.com also has a section on recipes, however, be careful to check the ingredient list against the food list, as not all of the published recipes are on the plan, no matter what anyone says.

There are nearly 100 recipes here and unfortunately, the electronic nature of the book does not allow us to make internal links in the middle of the book. You can, however, bookmark your favorites, or jump to them from the table of contents. There is even a recipe for breadsticks at the end.

LEGEND OF MEASUREMENT ABBREVIATIONS

teaspoon	tsp or t
tablespoon	tbsp or T
cup	c
gram	g
ounce	oz

SPICES and STOCKS

Greek Seasoning Mix

2 tsp (t) oregano
1 1/2 t onion powder
1 1/2 t garlic powder
1 t salt
1 t black pepper
1 t parsley
1 t basil
1/2 t cinnamon
1/2 t nutmeg
1/2 t thyme

Grind spices in food processor or coffee grinder.
Store in air-tight container.

Onion Soup Mix

1/2 c dehydrated minced onion
1 tbs (T) onion powder
1/2 t celery seed

Combine all ingredients.
Store in air-tight container.

TIP: This is wonderful to use dry in your ground steak for hamburgers, etc. It's an easy way to perk it up.

Mock Shake 'n Bake

1/2 c minced dehydrated onions
1/4 t coriander
1/4 t thyme
1/4 t red pepper flakes
1/8 t oregano
1/8 t paprika
1/8 t black pepper
1/8 t salt

Place all ingredients in food processor or coffee grinder.
Grind to a powder.
Store in air-tight container.

TIP: Use this as coating on your meat before you cook it. Dampen meat, then coat. This is great on chicken, fish, shrimp, even steakburgers.

This yields several portions.

Taco Seasoning

1 T chili powder
2 t onion powder
1 t ground cumin
1 t garlic powder
1 t paprika
1 t ground oregano

Mix ingredients & store in air-tight container.

Emeril's "Southwest Spice"

2 T chili powder
1 T dried oregano
2 T paprika
1 T ground coriander
1 T garlic powder
1 T salt
2 t ground cumin
1 t black pepper
1 t cayenne pepper
1 t ground red pepper

Combine all ingredients thoroughly and store in an airtight container.

Indian Curry Seasoning

1 T turmeric
1 T coriander
2 t paprika
1 t pepper
1 t cumin
1 t ginger
1/2 t cloves
1/2 t celery seed
1/2 t cayenne

Mix & store in air-tight container.

Seafood Seasoning

1 T ground bay leaves
2½ t celery seed
1½ t dry mustard
1½ t black pepper
¾ t ground nutmeg
½ t ground cloves
½ t ground ginger
½ t paprika

½ t red pepper
¼ t ground cardamom
¼ t ground mace

Mix all ingredients & store in an airtight container.

Caribbean Chicken Rub

1 T parsley
1 t cumin
1 t chili powder
1/2 t black pepper
1/2 t allspice
1/4 t cinnamon

This amount makes enough for 2 servings of chicken, shake in a Ziploc® bag. Let it sit for 20 mins in refrigerator before grilling/baking/broiling. Freeze the extra portion.

BBQ Rub

2 T paprika
1 T granulated sugar substitute
1 T ground cumin
1 T black pepper
1 T chili powder

Mix & store in air-tight container/-Ziploc® bag.

Marinara Sauce

tomato
water
 basil
parsley
onion powder
garlic (fresh minced)
salt
pepper

Fill small saucepan with a few cups of water & bring to boil.

Score skin of tomato in a few places with serrated knife.

Blanch tomato in the boiling water for 1-2 mins.

Immediately transfer tomato to ice water to cool and discard boiling water.

Remove skin of tomato and discard skin.

Preheat small <u>non-stick</u> saucepan over MED-HI heat.

If want chunky sauce, crush tomato with your hands in saucepan (discard stem). If you prefer smoother sauce, puree tomato in blender or food processor then add to pan.

Add garlic, onion powder, salt, pepper.

Bring to low boil, then immediately reduce heat to low, cover & simmer for 15 mins, stirring often to keep tomato from sticking.

Turn heat up to MED.

Add parsley, more garlic, and basil.

Cook 5-10 more minutes, stirring constantly. While cooking, start adding water 1T at a time until it reaches your desired consistency. I usually end up adding 3-4T of water.

Easy Homemade Broth

100g chicken (you can add more chicken - you just need to track your portions)
parsley
onion powder
garlic
thyme
rosemary
oregano
basil
bay leaf
salt
black pepper

Fill saucepan 3/4 full with water.

Bring to boil.

Add chicken and seasonings.

Boil for 20 mins.

Remove boiled chicken & serve or refrigerate and save for later.

Strain out bay leaf & seasonings.
Let broth cool to room temperature.
Skim fat off surface (if any).
Refrigerate broth.
Once cold, skim the rest of the fat from the top (if any).
Store in refrigerator or freeze for later use.

TIP: freeze the broth in ice cube trays after cooling and skimming all fat. Then after they freeze, place the cubes of broth in a freezer bag. This makes for easy use when 'frying' up shrimp, chicken, etc. Just toss a broth cube into a pan and let it melt then add your meat, etc.

SOUPS

Effortless Cream of Chicken Soup

100g cooked chicken
celery (allowed amount)
1-2 c broth (see broth recipe in stocks)
3 cloves garlic
1 T dehydrated minced onion
1/2 t parsley
1/2 t basil
ground white pepper (to taste)
salt (optional)

Preheat saucepan over MED-HI heat.
In food processor, combine all ingredients and pulse until reaches desired consistency.
Pour into saucepan and bring to boil.
Reduce heat to simmer, cover, and heat 20-30 mins.
Serve.

Green Onion Soup

• green onions (allowed amount)

- 2 c vegetable broth
- 1 t parsley
- 1 t SweetLeaf™ powder
- 1/2 t paprika
- 1/2 t salt
- 1/2 t dill
- 1/2 t thyme
- 1/8 t cayenne or red pepper flakes
- 1/8 t celery seed

Briefly steam the green onions until tender.
Preheat saucepan over MED heat.
Chop steamed green onions.
In a saucepan, sauté the green onions in a bit of vegetable broth for a couple of minutes, then add the parsley, SweetLeaf™ powder, paprika, salt, dill, thyme, celery seed, and cayenne. Saute 1-2 mins more.
Add remaining vegetable broth, reduce heat, cover and simmer 20-30 min.

Shrimp Stew

4 diced tomatoes
1 tsp Italian seasoning
1 tsp fennel seed
1 Tbsp diced garlic
1 diced onion
1 pound of peeled shrimp
Tabasco (or similar hot sauce) to taste

Grind together in a mini processor the seasoning, fennel seed, and garlic.
Add the spices onion, and 3/4 of the tomatoes to a saucepan with vegetable broth - or water.
Bring to a boil and simmer for 30 minutes.
Add the shrimp and the rest of the tomatoes and bring to a boil again.
Simmer until shrimp are cooked.
Add Tabasco to taste. 4 equal servings.

Chili

2 cups of chicken broth (I just use water)
3.5oz chicken or ground beef
1 cup or what you want of cabbage
1 tbl cumin
1.5 tbl chili seasoning
1 tbs minced onion
few pinches of onion powder
few pinches of garlic powder
diced tomatoes 1/2 cup
fresh garlic if you want.

Cook your chicken on stove with some water or broth cubes.
Add spices and all the rest of the ingredients
let simmer low of 20-30 min.

Spicy Cabbage Soup

3 cups shredded cabbage
½ tspn ground pepper
1 Tbsn Cajun spice (see spice section)
1 Tbsn Onion powder

Boil cabbage in chicken 4 cups chicken broth for 20 min
Add spices, cover and simmer for 15 more
Serve

Cinnamon Curry Chicken Soup

100g chicken - cubed
diced onion (allowed amount)
2 c broth
3 cloves minced garlic
1/2 t curry powder
1/4 t cinnamon
1/4 t pumpkin pie spice
salt/black pepper to taste

In saucepan, combine all ingredients.
Bring to a boil.
Reduce heat, cover, and simmer 45 mins.

The chicken can go straight from the freezer to the saucepan or crockpot on this one. If frozen, I place the breast in whole, and then when the soup is finished, I cube or shred the chicken. Very flavorful!

Lemon Chicken Soup

100g cooked chicken breast (diced or shredded)
chopped spinach (allowed amount)
2-3 c broth (see stock section for recipe)
Juice of 1 lemon
1 t thyme
sea salt to taste
ground white pepper to taste

Preheat saucepan over MED heat.
Combine all ingredients.
Bring to a boil, then simmer 20 mins.
Serve.

This is an easy way to use up that boiled chicken you used to make your broth. You can even make this in the crockpot using uncooked or frozen chicken cut into cubes.

Fish Soup

100g fish or seafood of choice
1 chopped tomato
2 c broth
2-3 cloves minced garlic

1 bay leaf
1 t dehydrated minced onion
1 t parsley
1/4 t oregano
1/4 t basil
1/8 t rosemary
1/8 t fennel seeds
salt/pepper to taste
Tabasco

Combine minced onion, parsley, oregano, basil, rosemary, and fennel seeds in food processor or grinder. Grind.
Add seasonings and all other ingredients except for seafood & Tabasco in saucepan.
Bring to a boil. Reduce heat, cover, and simmer for 30 mins.
Add fish and return to boil.
Reduce heat, cover, and simmer 5-15 mins.
Remove bay leaf.
Top with a few dashes of Tabasco just before serving.

Shrimp Hot & Sour Soup

100g shrimp
bok choy or asparagus
2 c broth
2 T rice vinegar
1 t SweetLeaf™ powder
1 t hot sauce
1/2 t white pepper
1/4 t ginger
crushed red pepper

In saucepan, combine broth, vinegar, SweetLeaf™, ginger, hot sauce and white pepper.
Bring to boil.
Reduce heat, cover, and simmer for 2-3 mins.
Add shrimp. Return to boil.
Add vegetable, cover, and simmer for 2-3 mins.

Sprinkle with crushed red pepper and serve

Spicy White Chili

100g cooked chicken breast, shredded
1-4 c broth
4 cloves minced garlic
1/2 t cumin
1/4 t oregano
1/4 t red pepper flakes
1/8 t ground cloves
Tabasco or hot sauce to taste

Preheat pot over MED-HI heat.
Add all ingredients except for Tabasco/hot sauce.
Bring to a boil then reduce heat to simmer, cover, & cook 30 mins.
Add Tabasco or hot sauce right before serving.

TIP: This is also great fixed in a small crockpot. Toss everything in and put it on while you're out and come back to great tasting dinner! If using the crockpot, you can use cut up uncooked chicken (even frozen!). Feel free to add your allowed vegetable to this as well - like chopped onion.

Meatball Soup

1 serving meatballs (see recipe in Entrée section)
2-3 c beef or chicken broth (see recipe in stock section
100g-200g bok choy, onion, or cabbage
fresh chopped cilantro
seasonings to taste

In saucepan, bring broth to boil.
Feel free to add any seasonings you like to taste (oregano, basil, pepper, garlic, etc). I'll usually add in some hot sauce or Tabasco as well.

Add cooked meatballs, vegetable choice.
Cover & simmer 20-30 minutes or until vegetables reach desired tenderness.
Top with fresh chopped cilantro.
Serve.

French Onion Soup

1 onion, thinly sliced
2 c beef broth
3-4 cloves minced garlic
1/2 t SweetLeaf™ powder
1/4 t black pepper

Preheat non-stick saucepan over MED heat.
Place onions and garlic in pan and cook uncovered 5-10 mins.
Stir in SweetLeaf™ powder
Cook 10-15 mins until onions are caramelized.
Add beef broth & bring to boil.
Reduce heat to simmer, cover, and cook 20 mins.
Add black pepper.
Serve.

Mexican Chicken Soup

100g cooked chicken, shredded into bite-sized pieces
3-4 cloves minced garlic
1 t cumin
1/2 t onion powder
1/2 t chili powder
1/2 t cayenne (use less if you don't want it as spicy)
diced tomato
2-3 c broth (see spices and stocks for recipe)
1/4 c fresh chopped cilantro (optional)

Preheat pot over medium-high heat.

Add garlic, and cook for 3-5 minutes. (Heat until you see little bubbles around the garlic.)
Use a bit of your broth to keep garlic from sticking to the pot, if necessary.
Add tomatoes, chicken broth, and onion powder, cumin, chili powder, and cayenne.
Bring to a boil.
Reduce heat to a simmer, and add chicken.
Simmer for 20 minutes.
Stir in cilantro, and simmer for 5 minutes more.

Tomato Soup

1 tomato
1 clove minced garlic
1/2 c water
3/4 t basil (vary to taste)
1/2 t onion powder
salt
black pepper

Preheat broiler.
Cut tomato(es) in half.
Place tomato(es) on nonstick baking sheet. Flat side down.
Broil for 5-10 mins, or until the skins are blistered and blackened.
Let cool, then remove skins & seeds.
In a medium sized saucepan, heat 1/4 c water over medium heat.
Add onion powder & cook for 5 minutes.
Add garlic & cook for 2 more minutes.
While that's cooking, place tomato(es) in a blender or food processor and puree until smooth.
Stir tomato puree into saucepan and add the rest of your water (1/4 c).
Bring to a boil then reduce to simmer for 5 minutes.
Stir in basil and season with salt & pepper.

Radish Soup

radishes (sliced or coarsely chopped - however you prefer)
1-2 cloves minced garlic
2 c stock
Salt
pepper

Combine all ingredients in saucepan.
Bring to a boil.
Reduce heat and simmer 10-15 mins.
Serve immediately.

Cinnamon Curry Chicken Soup

100g chicken - cubed
diced onion (allowed amount)
2 c broth
3 cloves minced garlic
1/2 t curry powder
1/4 t cinnamon
1/4 t pumpkin pie spice
salt/black pepper to taste

In saucepan, combine all ingredients.
Bring to a boil.
Reduce heat, cover, and simmer 45 mins.

Entrées

BEEF

Mini Meatloaf

100g ground steak
1/2 t milk or BBQ sauce (see spice recipes)
1 grissini (ground into powder)
2-3 cloves minced garlic
1/2 t dehydrated minced onion
1/2 t spicy mustard
1/4 t allspice
1/8 t sage
salt/pepper to taste
Any additional seasonings you like

Preheat oven to 350.
In small bowl, combine all ingredients and form into a small meatloaf.
Place in glass dish, cover, and bake 25-30 mins.
Uncover dish, add BBQ sauce or homemade-sugar-free ketchup to top, and bake 5-10 additional mins.
Serve immediately with a bit more of BBQ sauce or homemade sugar-free ketchup for dipping.

Meat in Tomato Sauce

100 g of lean hamburger, chicken, shrimp, fish (or whatever meat you would like to eat)
1 large or 2 small tomatoes
1/4 tsp. of garlic salt
1/4 tsp. onion salt
1/4 tsp. Italian Seasoning (make sure it has 0 carbs)

First, slice up your tomato(es) and put them into a sauce pan to sauté on medium for about 5 minutes. While they are being heated, occasionally
smash the tomatoes with a spoon. While the tomatoes are heating, put your meat on the grill.
When your tomatoes are heated and soft, they should have the consistency of THICK spaghetti sauce (or whatever consistency you prefer).
After the hamburger is properly cooked, mix it together with the tomatoes. Add in your spices, stir, and enjoy!

Crockpot Roast

100g steak
onion soup mix (see soup recipe)
1 c beef broth (see soup recipe)
black pepper to taste

Add steak to crockpot.
Cover with remaining ingredients.
Cook for several hours until reaches desired doneness.
Serve.

Rosemary Garlic Steak

100g steak
1 T rice vinegar
1 T rosemary
1 t garlic paste (3-5 cloves minced)
1/2 t crushed red pepper

In small dish, add rice vinegar. Add steak and coat.
In small bowl, combine rosemary, garlic, red pepper. Rub on both sides of steak.
Place steak in small dish, cover, and refrigerate 4 hours - overnight.
Grill to desired doneness.

Thai Cucumber Beef Salad

100g steak
1 t mild Tabasco or red pepper flakes
2-3 cloves minced garlic or 1 t garlic paste
1/4 t ground white pepper
2-3 T water
100g cucumber
half lemon
chopped cilantro

1. Peel, seed and slice cucumber.
2. In small dish, combine cucumber, juice of 1/2 lemon, and chopped cilantro. Toss.
3. Cover & refrigerate to marinate while preparing the rest of the dish.
4. Preheat pan over MED-HI heat.
5. Slice steak into very thin slices.
6. In small bowl, place steak, mild Tabasco, garlic, and white pepper. Be sure to coat steak well.
7. Place steak in pan with water.
8. Stir fry for 2-5 mins depending on how you like your steak cooked.
9. Serve immediately while hot over cold cucumbers.

NOTE: This is a flavor party for the taste buds!

French Dip

100g sliced cooked steak
1/2 onion sliced into rings
1 c beef broth (see soup recipe)
2 cloves minced garlic
1/2 t thyme
1/2 t pepper

Preheat pan over MED heat.
Add onions and garlic. Cook 5-10 mins until tender.
Add broth, thyme, and pepper. Bring to boil.
Reduce heat & simmer 5-10 mins.
Add steak and return to boil.
Reduce heat & simmer 5-10 mins.
Serve steak & onions with the au jus.

Steak (or Chicken) and Tomato

100g steak (or chicken)
tomato (diced)
2-3 cloves minced garlic
1 t oregano
1 t basil
1/4 t chili powder
black pepper

1. Preheat oven to 350.
2. Place 1/2 of the diced tomato in casserole dish.
3. Add meat on top of tomato and top with minced garlic.
4. In small bowl, toss the rest of tomato with the oregano, basil, chili powder, and black pepper. Place on top of steak.
5. Cover tightly with aluminum foil or with lid.
6. Bake 45-60 mins.

TIP: If using chicken, sear each side for a minute or two in a frying pan with a dash of salt/pepper (until just browned). Then follow with same steps as above.

Chili

100g ground steak
1 tomato
1/2 c water or broth, (see broth recipe)
3-4 cloves minced garlic

Seasonings (to taste):
1/2 t onion powder
1/2 t oregano
1/4 t cumin
1/4 t black pepper
1/4 t cayenne
1/4 t basil
1/4 t thyme

Preheat pan over MED heat.
Add minced garlic and 1 T of the water/broth to pan.
Sauté 2-3 minutes. Be sure not to burn the garlic. Add more water/broth as necessary.
Increase heat to MED-HI.
Add ground steak and sauté until brown - about 5 minutes.
Add all seasonings and cook an additional 3 minutes.
Continue to add more water/broth as necessary.
While that is cooking dice 1/2 of tomato and place other 1/2 in food processor or blender to puree.
Mix in tomatoes, puree, and rest of broth.
Turn heat down to MED-LO and simmer until it reaches desired consistency.

Meat Balls

100g steak (ground into hamburger)
1 grissini (ground into powder)
1 T milk
parsley

onion powder
basil
oregano
garlic
salt
pepper

Preheat oven to 425.
In bowl, combine all ingredients.
Form into 1" meatballs (makes about 6-7).
Place in baking dish or non-stick baking sheet and cook 10 minutes turning halfway through cooking time.

These are great to make in a batch, and freeze. Mark the bag to indicate how many are in a serving, and it is a quick, flavorful protein serving when time is short.

CHICKEN

Baked Cajun Chicken

100g chicken
1/2 T milk
1/2 t Cajun seasoning (see spice section)

Preheat oven to 350.
In small dish, coat both sides of chicken with milk.
Place chicken in glass baking dish.
Sprinkle top with Cajun seasoning.
Bake uncovered 20-30 mins until chicken is no longer pink.
Add Tabasco for more spice

Breaded Chicken Cutlets

100g chicken

1 grissini (ground into powder)
1/2 c homemade chicken broth
1/4 t garlic powder
1/4 t paprika
1/4 t poultry seasoning (optional)
1/4 t cayenne (use less if you want them less spicy)
salt/pepper to taste

Preheat pan over MED heat.
In small dish, combine grissini powder, garlic powder, paprika, poultry seasoning, cayenne, and salt/pepper. (You could also use Ziploc bag.)
Add chicken to seasonings and fully coat.
Add half of broth and chicken to pan.
Cook for approx. 3-4 mins each side depending on thickness of chicken. Keep adding more broth as it cooks off.
Serve immediately.

Fried Chicken Tenders

100g chicken
1 T milk
1 grissini
Seasonings (salt, pepper, paprika, ground red pepper, garlic powder)

Preheat oven to 350.
Slice chicken breast into 3 tenders.
In small bowl, mix milk and any seasonings you prefer.
Grind grissini in food processor until it is a powder. (I use my coffee grinder.)
Put grissini powder in a separate small bowl.
Add chicken to milk mixture and toss to coat well.
Then one at a time, place chicken in grissini powder and coat both sides of chicken.
Place chicken in glass baking dish and bake 30-40 mins, turning over halfway through.
In last 5 mins, turn on broiler and broil 2-3 mins each side.
Serve immediately.

Boneless Hot Wings

100g chicken breast tenders
1/4 c vinegar
1/4 c water
1-2 T cayenne pepper
1-2 T chili powder (adjust as needed)

In small bowl, mix vinegar, water, and cayenne pepper.
Add chicken to marinade and refrigerate for 1-2 hrs.
Preheat oven to 350.
Add chili powder to a small dish and dip chicken in chili powder.
Place on rack in baking pan.
Bake 15-20 mins turning halfway through.
Serve immediately with some homemade buffalo sauce or Hot Sauce.

Garlic Chicken

100g chicken400g chicken - 4 servings
diced onion
3-5 cloves garlic - unpeeled & left whole
juice of half lemon
black pepper to taste

Preheat oven to 350.
Heat non-stick saucepan over MED.
Add the onion. Stir constantly until tender. 5-10 mins.
Transfer onions to glass baking dish.
Place chicken atop onions.
Squeeze on lemon juice & sprinkle with pepper.
Place garlic around and on the chicken.
Cover tightly either with lid or aluminum foil.
Cook for 30-45 mins or until chicken is no longer pink.

Lemon Rosemary Chicken

100g chicken
half lemon
1/2 t rosemary
1/4 t pepper
1-2 cloves minced garlic

Heat non-stick pan over MED-HI heat.
In small bowl, grate lemon peel.
Add lemon juice, rosemary, pepper, and garlic.
Toss in chicken.
Place chicken in skillet. Cook 5 mins brushing with remaining juice mixture.
Turn over chicken and cook 5 more mins or until juices run clear.

Lemon Mustard Broiled Chicken

100g chicken
juice of 1/2 lemon
1 T spicy mustard
1/2 t black pepper
1/2 t oregano
1/4 t cayenne pepper

Preheat broiler.
Broil 1 side of chicken 5-10 mins until slightly browned.
In small bowl, add the rest of the ingredients and mix well.
Spoon mixture onto chicken. Flip over and coat other side.
Broil uncooked side 5-10 mins or until no longer pink.

Blackened Chicken Salad

100g chicken tenders
1 t paprika
1/2 t onion powder
1/2 t garlic powder

1/4 t oregano
1/4 t thyme
1/4 t white pepper
1/4 t black pepper
1/4 t ground red pepper
spinach or salad greens (as allowed)

Combine all spices and rub on chicken.
Grill until no longer pink.
Serve over spinach or salad greens.

Kung Pao Chicken

100g chicken - cut into chunks
chopped onion (allowed amount)
1-2 t mild tobacco sauce
red pepper flakes (optional)
Half cup vinegar

Seasoning
Mash together in small bowl:

3 cloves minced garlic
1-2 t fresh minced ginger root

Sauce
Stir together in small bowl:
1/2 c broth (see broth recipe)
1 t rice vinegar

In small dish, combine ½ cup vinegar & chicken.
Refrigerate 30 mins - 1 hour.
Preheat non-stick pan over MED-HI heat.
Cook chicken 5-7 mins, browning on all sides.
Add mild tobacco and cook 1-3 additional mins.
Remove chicken from pan and set aside.
Add onion to pan and cook until tender.
Stir seasoning mixture in with onions. Cook 1-3 mins.

Add sauce mixture to pan. Cook 1-3 mins.
Re-add chicken to pan. Stir. Cook 1-3 mins.
Top with a few dashes of red pepper flakes (optional).
Serve.

FISH

Curried Broiled Fish

100g fish
1 sliced tomato
1/2 lemon
1/2-1 t curry seasoning (see spice section)

Preheat broiler.
Place fish on broiler rack.
Squeeze 1/2 lemon over fish.
Sprinkle with curry seasoning.
Place tomato slices on top of fish.
Broil 8"-10" away from broiler for 10-15 mins until tomato starts to blacken.
Serve.

Wasabi Whitefish

100g whitefish
1 T spicy mustard
1/2-1 t wasabi powder (the more you add the spicier it will be)
1/2 t ginger

In small dish, combine spicy mustard and wasabi powder. Mix in ginger.
Add fish to dish and coat.
Let stand for 15-30 mins.
Grill 4-5 mins on the grill until fish flakes. Or you can broil for 5-10 mins depending on thickness of fish.

Ginger Mahi-Mahi

100g mahi-mahi (or any whitefish)
1 t minced garlic
1 t ginger
black pepper (to taste)
sliced tomato (however much you're allowed)
juice of ½ or 1 lemon

Place mahi-mahi on top of a large sheet non-stick aluminum foil.
Cover with garlic, ginger, and pepper.
Place tomatoes on top of seasoned fish.
Top with squeezed lemon juice.
Close up aluminum foil into a "pouch" so that the top and ends are sealed.
Bake at 350 for 10-20 mins (depending on thickness) or until fish flakes.

Red Snapper w/ Fennel

100g red snapper (or any whitefish)
fennel (weigh out your portion) - cut into 1" pieces
lemon
2 t fresh ginger
1 t pepper

Place fish in shallow dish.
Squeeze lemon juice in small bowl.
Stir in ginger & pepper.
Pour on fish and marinate in refrigerator for 2 hours.
Remove fish from marinade and place in glass baking dish.
Place chopped fennel on top.
Cover dish with lid or aluminum foil and bake at 350 for 20-30 mins or until fish flakes.

Spicy Cilantro Whitefish

100g fish
juice of 1/2 lemon

1/2 c cilantro - pack measuring cup with cilantro leaves (remove from stems)
3 cloves minced garlic
1 Tmild hot sauce
1 T water (as needed)
red pepper flakes (optional)

Preheat oven to 400.
In food processor, combine cilantro, garlic, and mild hot sauce.
Start to pulse and add water as necessary until reaches desired consistency.
Place fish in baking dish or non-stick baking sheet.
Squeeze on fresh lemon juice, then top with cilantro mix.
Bake for 10-20 mins depending on thickness, until fish flakes.
Top with red pepper flakes (optional).
Serve.

Teriyaki Fish

100g whitefish
1 T rice vinegar (be sure to read the ingredients so that it includes NO sugar)
2 cloves minced garlic
1 t ginger

Mix rice vinegar, garlic, and ginger in a Ziploc® bag or dish with lid.
Place whitefish in marinade and coat.
Seal and refrigerate for 30 mins - 1 hr, turning once.
Discard marinade and pat fish slightly dry with a papertowel.
Grill 3-4 mins on the grill until fish flakes. Or you can broil for 5-10 mins depending on thickness of fish.

Creole Catfish

100g catfish (or any whitefish)
1 chopped tomato
1/2 c water
1 t minced onion
1-2 t Cajun Seasoning (see spices recipes)

Preheat pan over MED-HI heat.
Cut fish into bite size pieces.
Place fish in **Ziploc**® bag. Add minced onion & Cajun seasoning to coat.
Pan fry coated fish in pan with water.
Cook 3-4 mins. If all the water cooks off, add more as needed.
Add chopped tomato & stir fry for another 5-10 mins until tomatoes become tender and dish becomes more soupy.

Lemon Oregano Whitefish Packet w/ Asparagus

100g whitefish
asparagus (allowed amount)
juice of one lemon
1 t oregano
salt/pepper

Preheat the oven to 400F.
Snap off woody ends of asparagus and discard.
Tear off a large sheet of non-stick aluminum foil.
In the center of this sheet, place asparagus spears and sprinkle with salt/pepper.
Place whitefish on top of asparagus.
In small bowl, combine lemon juice & oregano, and pour over fish.
Fold up edges and completely seal packet on all sides.
Bake 10-20 mins, until fish flakes.
Serve.

Curried Broiled Fish

- 100g fish
- 1 sliced tomato
- 1/2 lemon
- 1/2-1 t curry seasoning (see spices recipe)

Preheat broiler.
Place fish on broiler rack.
Squeeze 1/2 lemon over fish.
Sprinkle with curry seasoning.
Place tomato slices on top of fish.
Broil 8"-10" away from broiler for 10-15 mins until tomato starts to blacken.
Serve.

NOTE: This includes both your meat and vegetable for this meal.

CRAB

Spicy Crab Cucumber Salad

- 100g crab - shredded
- cucumber - peeled, seeded, and julienned (allowed amount)
- 1/2 T rice vinegar
- 1/2-1 T spicy mustard
- 1/2-1 t wasabi powder
- grissini - coarsely ground

Combine rice vinegar, spicy mustard, and wasabi powder. Stir. Add remaining ingredients, toss & serve.

NOTE: This includes your meat, veggie, and grissini portion for this meal.

Crab Cakes

100g crab meat
1 grissini (ground into powder)
1 t parsley
1/2 t tarragon
1/2 t paprika
1/2 t lemon juice
1/4 t cayenne
1/4 t white pepper
1/4 t dry mustard
1/4 t seafood seasoning (optional)

Grind grissini into powder and place into small dish.
In bowl, combine crab meat and remaining ingredients. Mix well &
form into patties.
Coat each side of patty with grissini powder.
Brown in non-stick skillet over MED heat for 3 mins each side, or place
on George Foreman for 4-5 mins.
Serve immediately.

SHRIMP

Shrimp Stuffed Tomato

100g cooked shrimp
tomato(es) - allowed amount
juice of half lemon
1 T parsley (and any additional seasonings you like)
salt/pepper to taste
Tabasco (optional)

Place cooked shrimp in food processor. Pulse a few times to chop
up shrimp. Or, simply chop with sharp knife.
In small bowl, combine chopped shrimp, parsley, lemon juice, and
salt/pepper.
Cover and refrigerate 30 mins-1 hr.

When ready to serve, cut off top of tomato. Scoop out inside of tomato.

Chop & combine inside of tomato with shrimp mix. (You may discard seeds if you like.)

Fill tomato with shrimp mix.

Top with a couple dashes of Tabasco (optional) and serve.

TIP: This is great using baked fish as well.

Curry Shrimp

100g shrimp
onion - chopped (allowed amount)
1 t garlic paste (3-4 cloves minced)
1/8 c water
1/2 t curry powder
1/4 t cumin
salt/black pepper (to taste)

Preheat pan over MED heat.
Add onion and garlic. Cook until translucent. 5-10 mins.
Add shrimp, seasonings, and water. Mix & stir fry until cooked through.
Serve.

Garlic Shrimp

100g shrimp (peeled & deveined)
4-6 cloves minced garlic or 1-2 t garlic paste
1/2 c broth (see soup section for recipe)
1/2 t parsley
1/8 t dried thyme
1/8 t crushed red pepper
1 bay leaf

Heat nonstick pan over MED-HI heat.
Mix 1 T of the broth with red pepper, minced garlic, and bay leaf. Add to pan.
Cook less than a minute. Be sure not to burn the garlic.
Add shrimp. Cook 3 minutes.
Remove shrimp from pan.
Add the remainder of the 1/2 c broth, parsley, & thyme. Bring to a boil. Cook for 1-2 mins until reduced by half.
Return shrimp to pan & toss to coat.
Discard bay leaf & serve.

Shrimp Fried "Rice"

100g shrimp
200g cabbage
4 T homemade broth (see soup section for recipe)
1/2 t onion powder
1/2 t garlic powder (or use fresh minced, if available)
black pepper (to taste)
red pepper flakes (optional)

Preheat pan over MED-HI heat.
Finely shred cabbage in food processor.
Add cabbage, 2 T broth to pan.
Stir fry for 2-3 minutes just until slightly tender.
Remove cabbage and place on serving dish. Sprinkle with fresh black pepper.
Turn heat down to MED.
Add shrimp, 2 T broth, onion powder, garlic,
Stir fry shrimp until they curl up & turn pink.
Sprinkle with red pepper flakes. (optional)
Serve immediately over cabbage.

Don't expect the cabbage to taste like rice. But it has a great crunch and tenderness all at the same time, and goes really great with the shrimp. Really filling and tasty. Enjoy!

Boiled Shrimp

100g shrimp
2-3 c water (enough to cover shrimp in pan)
1/4 c apple cider vinegar
2 T seafood seasoning (see seasoning section)

Add water, apple cider vinegar, seafood seasoning and shrimp to saucepan over MED-HI heat.
Let water come to slow boil. When shrimp start floating, remove from heat & drain.
Immediately place shrimp in ice water for 1 minute.
Drain & serve immediately or chill in refrigerator.

Shrimp & Asparagus Stir Fry

100g shrimp (shelled & deveined)
1-2 cloves minced garlic
asparagus (allowed amt)
1 T fresh ginger

Add shrimp, garlic, and ginger into pre-heated pan.
Stir fry for 3-5 mins. (If needed, add small amount of water.)
While that cooks, snap ends off of asparagus. Cut asparagus into 2" pieces.
Remove shrimp from pan and add asparagus.
Stir fry for 2-3 mins.
Re-add shrimp to pan and heat for 1 minute to heat through.
Serve.

Cajun Shrimp Kebabs

100g shrimp
half lemon

fresh chopped parsley

Place shrimp in bowl & add 1T of Cajun Seasoning and toss to coat.
Put shrimp on skewers (if using wood skewers, remember to soak in water for at least 20 mins prior to use). You can also make kebabs with onion or tomato or any other veggie allowed on protocol.
Squeeze on lemon juice.
Grill or broil until cooked through.
Sprinkle with chopped parsley.
Serve.

Lemon Shrimp & Spinach

100g shrimp (peeled & deveined)
200g spinach (or amount allowed)
3T water
juice of 1 lemon (or 1/2 lemon if you like things less lemony)
4-5 cloves minced garlic
salt
black pepper

Preheat non-stick skillet over MED heat.
Add 3T water, garlic, and shrimp.
Cook 5 mins or until shrimp just turns pink. (Add water as necessary)
Squeeze in juice of 1 lemon.
Add spinach.
Toss in salt & pepper.
Cook uncovered until spinach wilts.
Serve.

VEGETABLES

Lemon Ginger Asparagus

asparagus (allowed amount)
1/2 c water
1/2 T fresh minced ginger root
3 cloves minced garlic
lemon zest
black pepper

1. Preheat pan over MED heat.
2. Snap off woody ends of asparagus spears & discard.
3. Snap spears into 2-3 pieces.
4. Add garlic & ginger to the pan & cook for 2-3 mins.
5. Add asparagus & water. Bring to a boil for 5 mins.
6. Remove asparagus and top with lemon rind & pepper.
7. Serve.

Cucumber Mint Salad

200g cucumber - sliced or diced
1 T vinegar (vary to taste - as I usually add about 3 T)
1 t black pepper
1 t minced garlic
1 t dried mint (I usually just snip up a bit of fresh mint that I have on hand)

Toss & mix all ingredients.
Cover.
Refrigerate for at least 1 hour.
Toss before serving.

Cucumber Salad

200g thinly sliced cucumber (or allowed amount)
1 T vinegar (to taste)
1 t dill
1/2 t SweetLeaf™ powder (or as needed)

black pepper

Combine all ingredients except cucumber & mix well.
Toss in cucumbers.
Cover & refrigerate. This tastes best if you wait at least one hour before serving.

Steamed Cabbage

cabbage (allowed amount)
juice of half lemon
1/2 t spicy mustard
salt/pepper (to taste)

Place cabbage in steamer. Cover and steam 5-10 mins, until slightly tender.
In small bowl, combine spicy mustard and lemon juice.
Place cabbage in bowl. Add lemon/mustard mix and toss.
Sprinkle with salt/pepper.
Serve immediately.

TIP: If you have no steamer available, simply place & cover a strainer/colander over a pot of boiling water.

Onion Rings

80g sliced onion rings
1 grissini
1 T skim milk (as allowed daily)
1/4 t cayenne pepper

1/4 t salt
1/4 t pepper

Preheat oven to 450.
In a small bowl, add milk, cayenne pepper, salt, pepper. Mix to make a batter.
Grind grissini in food processor until it is a powder. (I use my coffee grinder.)
Put grissini in a separate small bowl.
Place rings in batter bowl and toss to coat fully. (It's best to use your hands here to ensure you coat each ring.)
Let sit in batter 2-3 mins then toss again.
Dip each ring into the grissini powder by hand. I find it works best to do these one at a time, rolling the ring in the grissini coating instead of tossing or shaking it on.
Place on cookie sheet lined with non-stick aluminum foil.
Cook 6-7 mins. Then flip, cooking an additional 6-7 mins.
Serve immediately.

Roasted Asparagus

100g asparagus (or your allowed amount)
1-2 cloves minced garlic
1/2 t parsley
1/4 t oregano
black pepper (to taste)

Preheat oven to 400.
Trim asparagus.
Spread the spears on a sheet of non-stick aluminum foil.
Add the seasonings.
Wrap all ends of the foil up tightly to make a sealed 'pocket'.
Roast 15-20 minutes.

Sautéed Garlic & Greens

This makes quite a bit so be sure to weigh your portion prior to cooking and adjust recipe as needed.

6 cloves garlic, sliced
16 c (packed) stemmed and roughly chopped Swiss chard (about 5 large bunches)
squeeze of lemon
1/2 tsp salt

Heat garlic in large skillet over medium-low heat in a *non-stick* pan until garlic begins to turn golden, about 3 minutes. Transfer to small bowl and set aside.
Place greens and salt into the skillet. Using tongs, turn greens until wilted enough to fit in pan. Raise heat to medium and cover. Cook 7 to 10 minutes, tossing.
Transfer greens to a colander to drain. Return greens to pan and toss with reserved garlic.
Squeeze with lemon just before serving.
Refrigerate leftover greens in an airtight container for up to 3 days.

Baked Radishes Chips

200 grams of radishes – or allowed amount
sea or kosher salt
dried rosemary

Slice radishes, and place on baking paper on pan. Toss until well coated. Sprinkle with crushed dried rosemary and sea or kosher salt, and bake at 325 until they begin to turn brown.

Radish Hash

About 15 radishes
1 tspn onion powder
1 protein portion
Chicken broth (see soup section for recipe)
Salt, Pepper (curry if an Indian taste is desired)

Shred or chop your radishes. I chop mine with a slap-chop. Dice the onion.

Cover the bottom of a non-stick pan with chicken broth and heat it up.

Toss in your onions and radishes and protein.

Salt, pepper and spice them according to your tastes.

Toss and cook until onions and translucent and meat is cooked through.

Let sit and cook in pan and brown a bit. Serve up and enjoy!

FRUITS

Green Apple Slaw

1 green apple (mine was about 150g after coring)
juice from 1/2 small lemon (about 1 T)
granulated sugar substitute (to taste)
1/8 c cut fresh mint (optional)

Core, slice, and cut apple into slivers.

In bowl, add: apple, lemon juice, sugar substitute. Toss to mix.

Toss in fresh mint before serving.

Broiled Cinnamon Grapefruit

1/2 grapefruit
cinnamon to taste (optional)
SweetLeaf™ powder as needed

Take a knife around the inside peel of the grapefruit so that it cuts out the grapefruit from the peel. (I usually have to use my fingers after this to pull the grapefruit out.)

Separate the sections and place in a bowl. (It's best if the grapefruit is really juicy. If it's not, sprinkle with a bit of water to moisten.)

Sprinkle with SweetLeaf™ powder and cinnamon.

Toss, then place back into grapefruit peel.

Broil for about 3-5 mins until caramelized.

DESSERTS

Applesauce

This stuff is fantastic, on or off the program, it makes the house smell fantastic all day, and is a healthy all natural alternative to store bought, preserved applesauce.

1 apple
3 T water
cinnamon (optional)

Peel, core, and dice apple.
Place diced apple in mini-crockpot and add water.
Add cinnamon.
Cook at least two hours.
When finished, mash with spoon or fork, or place in blender to reach desired consistency.
Serve warm or refrigerate and serve cold.

Baked Apple

1 apple
cinnamon
ground cloves
ground nutmeg
water

Preheat oven to 350.
Core apple leaving about 1" in bottom. Do NOT core all the way through.
Place apple in baking dish.
Fill apple with 1/4 t cinnamon, 1/8 t ground cloves, dash nutmeg, fill remaining space with water (about 2tsp)
Pour 1/2 c water, 1/2 t cinnamon, 1/4 t ground cloves, and 1/2 t nutmeg around apple in the baking dish.
Bake for 45 mins - 1 hour.
Serve immediately.

Apple Crisp

Filling:
1 apple
half small lemon
1 T water
½ t SweetLeaf™ powder

cinnamon

Preheat oven to 400.
Peel, core, and slice/chop apple.
Place apples in small baking dish.
Cover with juice of 1/2 small lemon, SweetLeaf™, water, and few dashes of cinnamon. Toss.

Topping:
1 grissini stick
1 t milk
1/2 t cinnamon
1/4 t nutmeg
1/4 t pumpkin pie spice

Grind grissini into a powder using food processor or coffee grinder. Add milk in 1/4 t increments. Slowly stir until mixture forms a slightly moist crumbly topping.
Sprinkle on top of apple filling.

Bake:

Cover dish and bake 20 mins.
Remove cover and broil 1-2 mins to crisp topping.
Serve immediately.
NOTE: This is really filling and tastes like apple pie!

Coffee Popsicles

1 cup coffee
few drops of vanilla stevia
popsicle molds

Pour coffee into popsicle molds and sweeten with 2-3 drops of stevia, depending on how large the mold is.

Put in freezer and let freeze completely. Then enjoy as a snack or dessert!

Berry Popsicles

Flavored SweetLeaf™ water in Chocolate Rasberry, Orange Cream or Berry

Popsicle molds
Few drops of food color

Mix water, SweetLeaf™and color to desired taste and look. A few drops goes a long way, you only need 2-3 drops of SweetLeaf™and 3-4 to make a strong color in 3 cups of water.
Pour flavored/colored water in molds and freeze.

Strawberry Sorbet

- Allotted amount of strawberries
- Juice of 1 lemon
- sugar substitute (as needed)
- water (if needed)

Freeze fresh strawberries about 1 hour. (or use frozen strawberries)
Blend fresh frozen strawberries, lemon juice & sugar substitute in blender until very well blended.
You can serve immediately or place in freezer to allow it to firm up even further.

When off the program, add extra fruits like berries or banana. It is a great healthy frozen treat.

DRINKS

V8™ alike

tomato (allowed amount)

juice of half lemon

1 t fresh cilantro, minced

1/2 t **SweetLeaf™** powder or 2 drops

1/4-1/2 t garlic paste (to taste) or 1 clove minced

1/4 t cumin

1/4 t sugar-free Worcestershire

1/8 t celery seed

salt/pepper (to taste)

Tabasco (to taste)

1. In blender, combine all ingredients and puree until reaches desired consistency.
2. Place in refrigerator until chilled or serve over ice.

Pumpkin Berry Mocha

coffee
1 T milk
1/2 t pumpkin pie spice (to taste)
chocolate raspberry stevia (to taste)

Place all ingredients in blender and blend until frothy. Serve immediately.
Don't like the Berry taste – try it with the Chocolate Liquid Stevia instead!

TIP: You can also add ice to blender to make this a pumpkin mocha frappucino.

Simple Frappucino

Cool Coffee
Vanilla Crème Liquid Stevia

Mix ingredients and freeze until mushy. Or, add ice and blend until desired consistency.

Chai Tea

1 lb tea mix
3-4 cups of your choice of tea, loose
3-5 sticks cinnamon, ground into smallish pieces
Handful of whole cardamom pods
8-10 cloves, crushed
An allspice (they look like teeny walnuts), grated
¼ tsp Whole black pepper – crushed or ground coarsely in a pepper grinder
2-3 tsp ground ginger (don't use fresh, it has too much moisture)
Optional: 2-3 chopped vanilla beans

Mix all ingredients together and store in an air tight container.

To make tea, place mixture in tea ball and pour boiling water over the tea ball, cover and let steep for 15-20 minutes. Flavour if desired with Vanilla or Vanilla cream, or English Toffee SweetLeaf™

drops. Enjoy!

Strawberry Spinach Smoothie
I was sceptical about this one, but it is not bad, and it is filling.

1 can Fresca or Diet 7up
1 cup fresh spinach
1 cup frozen strawberries

Blend soda and spinach well. Add berries and blend until smooth

Lemon Soda

> Soda water
> Lemon Stevia
> Ice
> Mint

Crush ice and mix all ingredients, drink right away, Garnish with mint.

Lemon Fizz

> Naturally carbonated water
> ½ tsp. of lemon juice
> 1-2 packets of Stevia to taste

Mix the lemon juice with the Stevia & add the carbonated water. The carbonation relieves the urge to have a Coke or other pop that is not allowed.

Additionally you can get root beer flavored Stevia and add that to the carbonated water and it really DOES taste like root beer if you can get over the odd fact that it is clear instead of brown-colored

Grissini Breadsticks

These breadsticks are allowed on the diet, but only a small portion. It is easiest to purchase them in the cracker section of the grocer, however, if you can't find them there, here is a recipe . This recipe makes five dozen sticks the correct size.......it is vital to make them no larger than this in order to be successful on the program.

Dough:
  1 T active dry yeast
  1 ½ cups lukewarm water
  3 Cups + 2T unbleached flour
  2/3 Cups semolina flour
  2 T unsalted butter, softened
  1T extra virgin olive oil
  1 T salt

For forming breadsticks
  ½ cup unbleached bread flour
  ½ cup semolina flour
  ½ t salt
  2 T extra virgin olive oil
  1 T water

To make dough:
  In a small bowl, sprinkle the yeast over ¼ cup of lukewarm water and let stand 2 minutes to soften
  Whisk with a fork to dissolve the yeast, and let stand 5 minutes to activate
  Combine the yeast-water mix, bread flour, semolina flour, butter, olive oil, salt and remaining 1 ¼ cups water. Mix with the dough hook of an automatic mixer on medium speed for about 10 minutes. To mix by hand, mix the dough with a wooden spoon, then knead by hand for 10 minutes.
  Shape the dough into a ball and place in an oiled bowl. Turn to coat the dough with the oil, cover the bowl with plastic wrap, and let the dough rise until doubled, about 1 hour.

For Shaping:
  Combine the bread flour, semolina flour and salt in a small bowl and stir to blend.
  In another small bowl, combine the olive oil and water.
  Lightly oil four heavy rimmed baking sheets (or bake in batches).
  Sprinkle the work surface thickly with the flour mixture. Turn the dough out into the work surface and flatten it with a rolling pin

into an 18x6 inch rectangle. If the dough feels to soft and slack to shape the breadsticks, transfer the dough to a floured sheet pan and place in the freezer for about 10 minutes to firm it up. Return it to the floured work surface before continuing.

Brush the surface of the rectangle with the oil-water mixture, then sprinkle generously with some of the flour mixture.

With a chef's knife (or pizza cutter), cut the dough into 6-inch by 1/4-inch strips, cutting just a few at a time.

With your hands, pick each strip up by the ends. The dough is so supple that it will elongate as you lift it. Allow each strip to become only as long as the baking sheet, then arrange them side by side on the baking sheet, close but not touching.

Let rise about 30 minutes. Preheat oven to 350°. Bake the breadsticks until caramel-brown all the way through (test by breaking one open), about 30 minutes. Cool on a rack.

Drop me a note if you actually make this one!

APPENDIX A – THE ORIGINAL PROTOCOL

Dr. Simeons' Original Protocol

What follows is a copy of the original protocol produced by Dr. Simeons, MD for the Salvator Mundi International Hospital in Rome. The original is not dated but the first appearance of it was in the early 1960's when it was published in the public domain. Since then it has been circulated without contest and has recently been widely distributed by a number of sources on the Internet. The protocol was written by a doctor, for other doctors, to instruct them on how to run the program at their hospitals and clinics. Other doctors have written similar works, but this appears to be the original treatise, open for public domain.

 The program outlined in this book deviates minimally from the original protocol. The differences are:

- This program is done at home rather than in a clinic or hospital.
- The HCG is administered by sublingual (under the tongue) drops rather than shots, although information for shots is included if you prefer.
- This program does not recommend stopping during menstruation. The original allowed it because in the '50s many women would not leave the house during 'that time of the month.'

- This program introduces SweetLeaf™ as a sweet substitute that was not available at the time the protocol was written.
- This program helps find a widely accepted 'fit' weight prior to starting as a goal; this information was not available when the original protocol was created.

Additions to the original protocol are added in [brackets] to distinguish from the original. Because the original has been published multiple times, there are several variations in spelling and typographical errors. I have attempted to eliminate these by comparing multiple copies and verifying minor constant differences. One more thing….there are misspellings, and what appear to be grammar errors…..most of them are the difference between English and American grammar, though some are just the author. This was written in Europe, and as such conforms to that standard. I've kept them, as this is an accurate reprint of the original.

Pounds & Inches

A NEW APPROACH TO OBESITY

By: A.T.W. Simeons, M.D.

SALVATOR MUNDI INTERANTIONAL HOSPITAL

00152 – ROME

VIALE MURA GIANICOLENSI, 77

FORWARD

This book discusses a new interpretation of the nature of obesity, and while it does not advocate yet another fancy slimming diet it does describe a method of treatment which has grown out of theoretical considerations based on clinical observation.

What I have to say is, in essence, the views distilled out of forty years of grappling with the fundamental problems of obesity, its causes, its symptoms, and its very nature. In these many years of specialized work, thousands of cases have passed through my hands and were carefully studied. Every new theory, every new method, every promising lead was considered, experimentally screened and critically evaluated as soon as it became known. But invariably the results were disappointing and lacking in uniformity.

I felt that we were merely nibbling at the fringe of a great problem, as, indeed, do most serious students of overweight. We have grown pretty sure that the tendency to accumulate Abnormal fat is a very definite metabolic disorder, much as is, for instance, diabetes. Yet the localization and the nature of this disorder remained a mystery. Every new approach seemed to lead into a blind alley, as though patients were told that they are fat because they eat too much, we believed that this is neither the whole truth nor the last word in the matter.

Refusing to be side-tracked by all to facile interpretation of obesity, I have always held that overeating is the result of the disorder, not its cause, and that we can make little headway until we can build for ourselves some sort of theoretical structure with which to explain the condition. Whether such a structure represents the truth is not important at this moment. What it must do is give us an intellectually satisfying interpretation of what is happening in the obese body. It must also be able to withstand the onslaught of all hitherto known clinical facts and furnish a hard background against which the results of treatment can be accurately assessed.

To me this requirement seems basic, and it has always been the center of my interest. In dealing with obese patients it became a habit to register and order every clinical experience as if it were an odd looking piece of a jig-saw puzzle. And then, as in a jig saw puzzle, little clusters of fragments began to form, though they seemed to fit in nowhere. As the years passed these clusters grew bigger and started to amalgamate until about sixteen years ago, a complete picture became dimly discernible. This picture was, and still is, dotted with gaps for which I cannot find the pieces, but I do now feel that a theoretical structure is visible as a whole.

With mounting experience, more and more facts seemed to fit snugly into the new framework, and then, when a treatment based on such speculations showed consistently satisfactory results, I was sure that some practical advance had been made, regardless of whether the theoretical interpretation of the results is correct or not.

The clinical results of the new treatment have been published in scientific journal and these reports have been generally well received by the profession, but the very nature of a scientific article does not permit the full presentation of new theoretical concepts n or is there room to discuss the finer points of technique and the reasons for observing them.

During the 16 years that have elapsed since I first published my findings, I have had many hundreds of inquiries from research institutes, doctors and patients. Hitherto I could only refer those interested to my scientific papers, though I realized that these did not contain sufficient information to enable doctors to conduct the new treatment satisfactorily. Those who tried were obliged to gain their own experience through the many trials and errors which I have long since overcome.

Doctors from all over the world have come to Italy to study the method, first hand in my clinic in the Salvator Mutidi International Hospital in Rome. For some of them the time they could spare has been too short to get a full grasp of the technique, and in any case the number of those whom I have been able to meet personally is small compared with the many requests for further detailed information which keep coming in. I have tried to keep up with these demands by correspondence, but the volume of this work has become unmanageable and that is one excuse for writing this book.

In dealing with a disorder in which the patient must take an active part in the treatment, it is , I believe, essential that he or she have an understanding of what is being done and why. Only then can there be intelligent cooperation between physician and patient. In order to avoid writing two books, one for the physician and another for the patient – I have tried to meet the requirements of both in a single book. This is a rather difficult enterprise in which I may not have succeeded. The expert will grumble about long-windedness while the lay-reader may occasionally have to look up an unfamiliar word in the glossary provided for him.

To make the text more readable I shall be unashamedly authoritative and avoid all the hedging and tentativeness with which it is customarily to express new scientific concepts grown out of clinical experience and not as yet confirmed by clear-cut laboratory experiments. Thus, when I make what reads like a factual statement, the professional reader may have to translate into clinical experience seems to suggest that such and such an observation might be tentatively explained by such and such a working hypothesis, requiring a vast amount of further research before the hypothesis can be considered a valid theory. If we can from the outset establish this is a mutually accepted convention, I hope to avoid being accused of speculative e exuberance.

Obesity a Disorder

As a basis for our discussion we postulate that obesity in all of its many forms is due to an abnormal functioning of some part of the body and that everyone of abnormally accumulated fat is always the result of the same disorder of certain regulatory mechanisms. The persons suffering from this particular disorder will get fat regardless of whether they eat excessively, normally or less than normal. A person who is free of the disorder will never get fat, even if he frequently over eats.

Those in whom the disorder is severe will accumulate fat very rapidly, those in whom it is moderate will gradually increase in weight and those in whom it is mild may be able to keep their excess weight stationary for long periods. In all these cases a loss of weight brought about by dieting, treatments with thyroid, appetite-reducing drugs, laxatives, violent exercise, massage, or baths is only temporary and will be rapidly regained as soon as the reducing regimen is relaxed. The reason is simply that none of these measures corrects the basic disorder.

While there are great variations in the severity of obesity, we shall consider all the different forms in both sexes and at all ages as always being due to the same disorder. Variations in form would then be partly a matter of degree, partly an inherited bodily constitution and partly the result of a secondary involvement of endocrine glands such as the pituitary, the thyroid, the adrenals or the sex glands. On the other hand, we postulate that no deficiency of any of these glands can ever directly produce the common disorder known as obesity.

If this reasoning is correct, it follows that a treatment aimed at curing the disorder must be equally effective in both sexes, at all ages and in all forms of obesity. Unless this is so, we are entitled to harbor grave doubts as to whether a given treatment corrects the underlying disorder. Moreover, any claim that the disorder has been corrected must be substantiated by the ability of the patient to eat normally of any food he pleases without regaining Abnormal fat after treatment. Only if these conditions are fulfilled can we legitimately speak of curing obesity rather than of reducing weight.

Our problem thus presents itself as an enquiry into the localization and the nature of the disorder which leads to obesity. The history of this enquiry is a long series of high hopes and bitter disappointments.

The History of Obesity

There was a time, not so long ago, when obesity was considered a sign of health and prosperity in man and of beauty, amorousness and fecundity in women. This attitude probably dates back to Neolithic times, about 8000 years ago; when for the first time in history of culture, man began to own property, domestic animals, arable land, houses pottery and metal tools. Before that, with the possible exception of some races such as the Hottentots, obesity was almost non-existent, as it still is in all wild animals and most primitive races.

Today obesity is extremely common among all civilized races, because a disposition to the disorder can be inherited. Wherever Abnormal fat was regarded as an asset, sexual selection tended to propagate the trait. It is only in very recent times that manifest obesity has lost some of its allure, though the cult of the outsized bust – always a sign of latent obesity – shows that the trend still lingers on.

The Significance of Regular Meals

In the early Neolithic times another change took place which may well account for the fact that today nearly all inherited dispositions sooner or later develop into manifest obesity. This change was the institution of regular meals. In pre-Neolithic times, man ate only when he was hungry and only as much as he required to still the pangs of hunger. Moreover, much of his food was raw and all of it was unrefined. He roasted his meat, but he did not boil it, as he had no pots, and what little he may have grubbed from the Earth and picked from the trees, he ate as he went along.

The whole structure of man's omnivorous digestive tract is, like that of an ape, rat or pig, adjusted to the continual nibbling of tidbits. It is not suited to occasional gorging as is for instance, the intestine of the carnivorous cat family. Thus the institution of regular meals, particularly of food rendered rapidly, placed a great burden on modern man's ability to cope with large quantities of food suddenly pouring into his system from the intestinal tract.

The institution of regular meals meant that man had to eat more than his body required at the moment of eating so as to tide him over until the next meal. Food rendered easily digestible suddenly flooded his body with nourishment of which he was in no need at the moment. Somehow, somewhere this surplus had to be stored.

Three Kinds of Fat

In the human body we can distinguish three kinds of fat. The first is the Structural fat which fills the gaps between various organs, a sort of packing material. Structural fat also performs such important functions as bedding the kidneys in soft elastic tissue, protecting the coronary arteries and keeping the skin smooth and taut. It also provides the springy cushion of hard fat under the bones of the feet, without which we would be unable to walk.

The second type of fat is normal reserves of fuel upon which the body can freely draw when the nutritional income from the intestinal tract is insufficient to meet the demand. Such normal reserves are localized all over the body. Fat is a substance which packs the highest caloric value into the smallest space so that normal reserves of fuel for muscular activity and maintenance of body temperature can be most economically stored in this form. Both these types of fat, structural and reserve, are normal and even if the body stocks them to capacity this can never be called obesity.

But there is a third type of fat which is entirely abnormal. It is the accumulation of such fat, and of such fat only, from which the overweight patient suffers. This Abnormal fat is also a potential reserve of fuel, but unlike the normal reserves it is not available to the body in a nutritional emergency. It is, so to speak, locked away in a fixed deposit and is not kept in a current account, as are the normal reserves.

When an obese patient tries to reduce by starving himself, he will first lose his Normal fat reserves. When these are exhausted he begins to burn up Structural fat, and only as a last resort will the body yield its abnormal reserves, though by that time the patient usually feels so weak and hungry that the diet is abandoned. It is just for this reason that obese patients complain that when they diet they lose the wrong fat. They feel famished and tired and their face becomes drawn and haggard, but their belly, hips, thighs and upper arms show little improvement. The fat they have come to detest stays on and the fat they need to cover their bones gets less and less. Their skin wrinkles and they look old and miserable. And that is one of the most frustrating and depressing experiences a human being can have.

Injustice to the Obese

When then obese patients are accused of cheating, gluttony, lack of will power, greed and sexual complexes, the strong become indignant and decided that modern medicine is a fraud and its representatives fools, while the weak just give up the struggle in despair. In either case the result is the same: a further gain in weight, resignation to an abominable fate and the resolution at least to live tolerably the short span allotted to them – a fig for doctors and insurance companies.

Obese patients only feel physically well as long as they are stationary or gaining weight. They may feel guilty, owing to the lethargy and indolence always associated with obesity. They may feel ashamed of what they have been led to believe is a lack of control. They may feel horrified by the appearance of their nude body and the tightness of their clothes. But they have a primitive feeling of animal content which turns to misery and suffering as soon as they make a resolute attempt to reduce. For this there are sound reasons.

In the first place, more caloric energy is required to keep a large body at a certain temperature than to heat a small body. Secondly the muscular effort of moving a heavy body is greater than in the case of a light body. The muscular effort consumes calories which must be provided by food. Thus, all other factors being equal, a fat person requires more food than a lean one. One might therefore reason that if a fat person eats only the additional food his body requires he should be able to keep his weight stationary. Yet every physician who has studied obese patients under rigorously controlled conditions knows that this is not true. Many obese patients actually gain weight on a diet which is calorically deficient for their basic needs. There must be some other mechanism at work.

Glandular Theories

At one time it was thought that this mechanism might be concerned with the sex glands. Such a connection was suggested by the fact that many juvenile obese patients show an under-development of the sex organs. The middle-age spread in men and the tendency of many women to put on weight in the menopause seemed to indicate ta casual connection between diminishing sex function and overweight. Yet, when highly active sex hormones became available, it was found that their administration had no affect whatsoever on obesity. The sex glands could therefore not be the seat of the disorder.

The Thyroid Gland

When it was discovered that the thyroid gland controls the rate at which body-fuel is consumed, it was thought that by administering thyroid gland to obese (sic) patients their Abnormal fat deposits could be burned up more rapidly. This too proved to be entirely disappointing, because as we now know, these abnormal deposits take no part in the body's energy-turnover - they are inaccessibly locked away. Thyroid medication merely forces the body to consume its Normal fat reserves, which are already depleted in obese patients, and then to break down structurally essential fat without touching the abnormal deposits. In this way a patient may be brought to the brink of starvation in spite of having a hundred pounds of fat to spare. Thus any weight- loss brought about by thyroid medication is always at the expense of fat of which the body is in dire need.

While the majority of obese patients have a perfectly normal thyroid gland and some even have an overactive thyroid, one also occasionally sees a case with a real thyroid deficiency. In such cases, treatment with thyroid brings about a small loss of weight, but this is not due to the loss of any Abnormal fat. It is entirely the result of the elimination of a mucoid substance, called myxedema, which the body accumulates when there is a marked primary thyroid deficiency. Moreover, patients suffering only from a severe lack of thyroid hormone never become obese in the true sense. Possibly also the observation that normal persons - though not the obese - lose weight rapidly when their thyroid becomes overactive may have contributed to the false notion that thyroid deficiency and obesity are connected. Much misunderstanding about the supposed role of the thyroid gland in obesity is still met with, and it is now really high time that thyroid preparations be once and for all struck off the list of remedies for obesity. This is particularly so because gibing thyroid gland to an obese patient whose thyroid is either normal or overactive, besides being useless, is decidedly dangerous.

The Pituitary Gland

The next gland to be falsely incriminated was the anterior lobe of the pituitary or hypothesis. This most important gland lies well protected in a bony capsule at the base of the skull. It has a vast number of functions in the body, among which is the regulation of all the other important endocrine glands. The fact that various signs of anterior pituitary deficiency are often associated with obesity raised the hope that the seat of the disorder might be in this gland. But although a large number of pituitary hormones have been isolated and many extracts of the gland prepared, not a single one or any combination of such factors proved to be of any value in the treatment of obesity. Quite recently, however, a fat-mobilizing factor has been found in pituitary glands but it is still too early to say whether this factor is destined to play a role in the treatment of obesity.

The Adrenals

Recently, a long series of brilliant discoveries concerning the working of the adrenal or suprarenal glands, small bodies which sit atop the kidneys, have created tremendous interest. This interest also turned to the problem of obesity when it was discovered that a condition which in some respects resembles a severe case of obesity-the so called Cushing's Syndrome-was caused by a glandular new-growth of the adrenals or by their excessive stimulation with ACTH, which is the pituitary hormone governing the activity of the outer rind or cortex of the adrenals.

When we learned that an abnormal stimulation of the adrenal cortex could produce signs that resemble true obesity, this knowledge furnished no practical means of treating obesity by decreasing the activity of the adrenal cortex. There is no evidence to suggest that in obesity there is any excess of adrenocortical activity; in fact, all the evidence points to the contrary. There seems to be rather a lack of adrenocortical function and a decrease in the secretion of ACTH from the anterior pituitary lobe.

So here again our search for the mechanism which produces obesity led us into a blind alley. Recently, many students of obesity have reverted to the nihilistic attitude that obesity is caused simply by overeating and that it can only be cured by under eating.

The Diencephalon or Hypothalamus

For those of us who refused to be discouraged there remained one slight hope. Buried deep down in the massive human brain there is a part which we have in common with all vertebrate animals the so-called diencephalon. It is a very primitive part of the brain and has in man been almost smothered by the huge masses of nervous tissue with which we think, reason and voluntarily move our body. The diencephalon is the part from which the central nervous system controls all the automatic animal functions of the body, such as breathing, the heart beat, digestion, sleep, sex, the urinary system, the autonomous or vegetative nervous system and via the pituitary the whole interplay of the endocrine glands. It was therefore not unreasonable to suppose that the complex operation of storing and issuing fuel to the body might also be controlled by the diencephalon. It has long been known that the content of sugar-another form of fuel-in the blood depends on a certain nervous center in the diencephalon. When this center is destroyed in laboratory animals they develop a condition rather similar to human stable diabetes. It has also long been known that the destruction of another diencephalic center produces a voracious appetite and a rapid gain in weight in animals which never get fat spontaneously.

The Fat- bank

Assuming that in many such a center controlling the movement of fat does exist, its function would have to be much like that of a bank. When the body assimilates from the intestinal tract more fuel than it needs at the moment, this surplus is deposited in what may be compared with a current account. Out of this account it can always be withdrawn as required. All Normal fat reserves are in such a current account, and it is probable that a diencephalic center manages the deposits and withdrawals.

When now, for reasons which will be discussed later, the deposits grow rapidly while small withdrawals become more frequent a point may be reached which goes beyond the diencephalon's banking capacity. Just as a banker might suggest to a wealthy client that instead of accumulating a large and unmanageable current account he should invest his surplus capital, the body appears to establish a fixed deposit into which all surplus funds go but from which they can no longer be withdrawn by the procedure used in a current account. In this way the diericephalic "fat-bank " frees itself from all work which goes beyond its normal banking capacity. The onset of obesity dates from the moment the diencephalon adopts this labor-saving ruse. Once a fixed deposit has been established the Normal fat reserves are held at a minimum, while every available surplus is locked away in the fixed deposit and is therefore taken out of normal circulation.

Three Basic Causes of Obesity

(1) The Inherited Factor

Assuming that there is a limit to the diencephalon's fat banking capacity, it follows that there are three basic ways in which obesity can become manifest. The first is that the fat-banking capacity is abnormally low from birth. Such a congenitally low diencephalic capacity would then represent the inherited factor in obesity. When this abnormal trait is markedly present, obesity will develop at an early age in spite of normal feeding; this could explain why among brothers and sisters eating the same food at the same table some become obese and others do not.

(2) Other Diencephalic Disorders

The second way in which obesity can become established is the lowering of a previously Normal fat-banking capacity owing to some other diencephalic disorder. It seems to be a general rule that when one of the many diencephalic centers is particularly overtaxed; it tries to increase its capacity at the expense of other centers.

In the menopause and after castration the hormones previously produced in the sex-glands no longer circulate in the body. In the presence of normally functioning sex-glands their hormones act as a brake on the secretion of the sex-gland stimulating hormones of the anterior pituitary. When this brake is removed the anterior pituitary enormously increases its output of these sex-gland stimulating hormones, though they are now no longer effective. In the absence of any response from the non-functioning or missing sex glands, there is nothing to stop the anterior pituitary from producing more and more of these hormones. This situation causes an excessive strain on the diericephalic center which controls the function of the anterior pituitary. In order to cope with this additional burden the center appears to draw more and more energy away from other centers, such as those concerned with emotional stability, the blood circulation (hot flushes) and other autonomous nervous regulations, particularly also from the not so vitally important fat-bank.

The so called stable type of diabetes involves the diencephalic blood sugar regulating center the diencephalon tries to meet this abnormal load by switching energy destined for the fat bank over to the sugar-regulating center, with the result that the fat-banking capacity is reduced to the point at which it is forced to establish a fixed deposit and thus initiate the disorder we call obesity. in this case one would have to consider the diabetes the primary cause of the obesity, but it is also possible that the process is reversed in the sense that a deficient or overworked fat-center draws energy from the sugar-center, in which case the obesity would be the cause of that type of diabetes in which the pancreas is not primarily involved. Finally, it is conceivable that in Cushing's Syndrome those symptoms which resemble obesity arc entirely due to the withdrawal of energy from the diencephalic fat-bank in order to make it available to the highly disturbed center which governs the anterior pituitary adrenocortical system.

Whether obesity is caused by a marked inherited deficiency of the fat-center or by some entirely different diencephalic regulatory disorder, its insurgence obviously has nothing to do with overeating and in either case obesity is certain to develop regardless of dietary restrictions. In these cases any enforced food deficit is made up from essential fat reserves and normal Structural fat, much to the disadvantage of the patient's general health.

(3) The Exhaustion of the Fat-bank

But there is still a third way in which obesity can become established, and that is when a presumably Normal fat-center is suddenly-the emphasis is on suddenly-called upon to deal with an enormous influx of food far in excess of momentary requirements. At first glance it does seem that here we have a straight-forward case of overeating being responsible for obesity, but on further analysis it soon becomes clear that the relation of cause and effect is not so simple. In the first place we are merely assuming that the capacity of the fat center is normal while it is possible and even probable that the only persons who have some inherited trait in this direction can become obese merely by overeating.

Secondly, in many of these cases the amount of loud eaten remains the same and it is only the consumption of fuel which is suddenly decreased, as when an athlete is confined to bed for many weeks with a broken bone or when a man leading a highly active life is suddenly tied to his desk in an office and to television at home. Similarly, when a person, grown up in a cold climate, is transferred to a tropical country and continues to eat as before, he may develop obesity because in the heat far less fuel is required to maintain the normal body temperature.

When a person suffers a long period of privation, be it due to chronic illness, poverty, famine or the exigencies of war, his diencephalic regulations adjust themselves to some extent to the low food intake. When then suddenly these conditions change and he is free to eat all the food he wants, this is liable to overwhelm his fat-regulating center. During the last war about 6000 grossly underfed Polish refugees who had spent harrowing years in Russia were transferred to a camp in India where they were well housed, given normal British army rations and some cash to buy a few extras. 'Within about three months 85% were suffering from obesity.

In a person eating coarse and unrefined food the digestion is slow and only a little nourishment at a time is assimilated from the intestinal tract. When such a person is suddenly able to obtain highly refined foods such as sugar, white flour, butter and oil these are so rapidly digested and assimilated that the rush of incoming fuel which occurs at every meal may eventually overpower the diecenphalic regulatory mechanisms and thus lead to obesity. This is commonly seen in the poor man who suddenly becomes rich enough to buy the more expensive refined foods, though his total caloric intake remains the same or is even less than before.

Psychological Aspects

Much has been written about the psychological aspects of obesity. Among its many functions the diencephalon is also the seat of our primitive animal instincts, and just as in an emergency it can switch energy from one center to another, so it seems to be able to transfer pressure from one instinct to another. Thus a lonely and unhappy person deprived of all emotional comfort and of all instinct gratification except the stilling of hunger and thirst can use these as outlets for pent up instinct pressure and so develop obesity. Yet once that has happened, no amount of psychotherapy or analysis, happiness, company or the gratification of other instincts will correct the condition.

Compulsive Eating

No end of injustice is done to obese patients by accusing them of compulsive eating, which is a form of diverted sex gratification. Most obese patients do not suffer from compulsive eating; they suffer genuine hunger-real, gnawing, torturing hunger-which has nothing whatever to do with compulsive eating. Even their sudden desire for sweets is merely the result of the experience that sweets, pastries and alcohol will most rapidly of all foods allay the pangs of hunger. This has nothing to do with diverted instincts.

On the other hand, compulsive eating does occur in some obese patients, particularly in girls in their late teens or early twenties. Fortunately from the obese patients' greater need for food, it comes on in attacks and is never associated with real hunger, a fact which is readily admitted by the patients. They only feel a feral desire to stuff. Two pounds of chocolates may be devoured in a few minutes; cold, greasy food from the refrigerator, stale bread, leftovers on stacked plates, almost anything edible is crammed down with terrifying speed and ferocity.

I have occasionally been able to watch such an attack without the patient's knowledge, and it is a frightening, ugly spectacle to behold, even if one does realize that mechanisms entirely beyond the patient's control are at work. A careful enquiry into what may have brought on such an attack almost invariably reveals that it is preceded by a strong unresolved sex-stimulation, the higher centers of the brain having blocked primitive diencephalic instinct gratification. The pressure is then let off through another primitive channel, which is oral gratification. In my experience the only thing that will cure this condition is uninhibited sex, a therapeutic procedure which is hardly ever feasible, for if it were, the patient would have adopted it without professional prompting, nor would this in any way correct the associated obesity. It would only raise new and often greater problems if used as a therapeutic measure.

Patients suffering from real compulsive eating are comparatively rare. In my practice they constitute about 1-2%. Treating them for obesity is a heartrending job. They do perfectly well between attacks, but a single bout occurring while under treatment may annul several weeks of therapy. Little wonder that such patients become discouraged. In these cases I have found that psychotherapy may make the patient fully understand the mechanism, but it does nothing to stop it. Perhaps society's growing sexual permissiveness will make compulsive eating even rarer.

Whether a patient is really suffering from compulsive eating or not is hard to decide before treatment because many obese patients think that their desire for food-to them unmotivated__ is due to compulsive eating, while all the time it is merely a greater need for food. The only way to find out is to treat such patients. Those that suffer from real compulsive eating continue to have such attacks, while those who are not compulsive eaters never get an attack during treatment.

Reluctance to Lose Weight

Some patients are deeply attached to their fat and cannot bear the thought of losing it. If they are intelligent, popular and successful in spite of their handicap, this is a source of pride. Some fat girls look upon their condition as a safeguard against erotic involvements, of which they are afraid. They work out a pattern of life in which their obesity plays a determining role and then become reluctant to upset this pattern and face a new kind of life which will be entirely different after their figure has become normal and often very attractive. They fear that people will like them -or be jealous-on account of their figure rather than he attracted by their intelligence or character only. Some have a feeling that reducing means giving up an almost cherished and intimate part of themselves. In many of these cases psychotherapy can be helpful, as it enables these patients to see the whole situation in the full light of consciousness An affectionate attachment to Abnormal fat is usually seen in patients who became obese in childhood, but this is not necessarily so. In all other cases the best psychotherapy can do in the usual treatment of obesity is to render the burden of hunger and never- ending dietary restrictions slightly more tolerable. Patients who have successfully established an erotic transfer to their psychiatrist are often better able to hear their suffering as a secret labor of love.

There are thus a large number of ways in which obesity can be initiated though the disorder itself is always due to the same mechanism, an inadequacy of the diencephalic fat-center and the laying down of abnormally fixed fat deposits in abnormal places. This means that once obesity has become established, it can no more be cured by eliminating those factors which brought it on than a fire can be extinguished by removing the cause of the conflagration. Thus a discussion of the various ways in which obesity can become established is useful from a preventative point of view, but it has no bearing on the treatment of the established condition. The elimination of factors which are clearly hastening the course of the disorder may slow down its progress or even halt it, but they can never correct it.

Not by Weight Alone

Weight alone is not a satisfactory criterion on by which to judge whether a person is suffering from the disorder we call obesity or not.

Every physician is familiar with the sylphlike lady who enters the consulting room and declares emphatically that she is getting horribly fat and wishes to reduce. Many an honest and sympathetic physician at once concludes that he is dealing with a "nut." If he is busy he will give her short shrift, but if he has time he will weigh her and show her tables to prove that she is actually underweight.

I have never yet seen or heard of such a lady being convinced by either procedure. The reason is that in my experience the lady is nearly always right and the doctor wrong. When such a patient is carefully examined one finds many signs of potential obesity, which is just about to become manifest as overweight. The patient distinctly feels that something is wrong with her, that a subtle change is taking place in her body, and this alarms her.

There are a number of signs and symptoms which are characteristic of obesity. In manifest obesity many and often all these signs and symptoms are present. In latent or just beginning cases some are always found, and it should be a rule that if two or more of the bodily signs are present the case must be regarded as one that needs immediate help.

Signs and Symptoms of Obesity

The bodily signs may be divided into such as have developed before puberty, indicating a strong inherited factor, and those which develop at the onset of manifest disorder. Early signs are a disproportionately large size of the two upper front teeth, the first incisor, or a dimple on both sides of the sacral bone just above the buttocks. When the arms are outstretched with the palms upward, the forearms appear sharply angled outward from the upper arms. The same applies to the lower extremities. The patient cannot bring his feet together without the knees overlapping; he is, in fact, knock-kneed.

The beginning accumulation of Abnormal fat shows as a little pad just below the nape of the neck, colloquially known as the Duchess' Hump. There is a triangular fatty bulge in front of the armpit when the arm is held against the body. When the skin is stretched by fat rapidly accumulating under it, it many split in the lower layers. When large and fresh, such tears are purple, but later they are transformed into white scar-tissue. Such striation, as it is called, commonly occurs on the abdomen of women during pregnancy, but m obesity it is frequently found on the breasts, the hips and occasionally on the shoulders. In many cases striation is so fine that the small white lines are only just visible. They are always a sure sign of obesity, and though this may be slight at the time of examination such patients can usually remember a period in their childhood when they were excessively chubby.

Another typical sign is a pad of fat on the insides of the knees, a spot where Normal fat reserves are never stored. There may be a fold of skin over the pubic area and another fold may stretch round both sides of the chest, where a loose roll of fat can be picked up between two fingers. In the male an excessive accumulation of fat in the breasts is always indicative, while in the female the breast is usually, but not necessarily, large. Obviously excessive fat on the abdomen, the hips, thighs, upper arms, chin and shoulders are characteristic, and it is important to remember that any number of these signs may be present in persons whose weight is statistically normal; particularly of they are dieting on their own with iron determination.

Common clinical symptoms which are indicative only in their association and in the frame of the whole clinical picture are: frequent headaches rheumatic pains without detectable bony abnormality; a feeling of laziness and lethargy, often both physical and mental and frequently associated with insomnia, the patients saying that all they want is to rest; the frightening feeling of being famished and sometimes weak with hunger two to three hours after a hearty meal and an irresistible yearning for sweets and starchy food which often overcomes the patient quite suddenly and is sometimes substituted by a desire for alcohol; constipation and a spastic or irritable colon are unusually common among the obese, and so are menstrual disorders.

Returning once more to our sylphlike lady, we can say that a combination of some of these symptoms with a few of the typical bodily signs is sufficient evidence to take her case seriously. A human figure, male or female, can only be judged in the nude; any opinion based on the dressed appearance can be quite fantastically wide off the mark, and I feel myself driven to the conclusion that apart from frankly psychotic patients such as cases of anorexia nervosa a <

morbid weight fixation > does not exist. I have yet to see a patient who continues, to complain after the figure has been rendered normal by adequate treatment.

The Emaciated Lady

I remember the case of a lady who was escorted into my consulting room while I was telephoning. She sat down in front of my desk, and when I looked up to greet her I saw the typical picture of advanced emaciation. Her dry skin hung loosely over the bones of her face, her neck was scrawny and collarbones and ribs stuck out from deep hollows. I immediately thought of cancer and decided to which of my colleagues at the hospital I would refer her. Indeed, I felt a little annoyed that my assistant had not explained to her that her case did not fall under my specialty. In answer to my query as to what I could do for her, she replied that she wanted to reduce. I tried to hide my surprise, but she must have noted a fleeting expression, for she smiled and said "I know that you think I'm mad, but just wait." With that she rose and came round to my side of the desk. Jutting out from a tiny waist she had enormous hips and thighs.

By using a technique which will presently be described, the Abnormal fat on her hips was transferred to the rest of her body emaciated by months of very severe dieting. At the end of a treatment lasting five weeks she, a small woman, had lost 8 inches round her hips, while her face looked fresh and florid, the ribs were no longer visible and her weight was the same to the ounce as it had been at the first consultation.

Fat but not Obese

While a person who is statistically underweight may still be suffering from the disorder which causes obesity, it is also possible for a person to be statistically overweight without suffering from obesity. For such persons weight is no problem, as they can gain or lose at will and experience no difficulty in reducing their caloric intake. They are masters of their weight, which the obese are not. Moreover, their excess fat shows no preference for certain typical regions of the body, as does the fat in all cases of obesity. Thus, the decision whether a borderline case is really suffering from obesity or not cannot be made merely by consulting weight tables.

The Treatment of Obesity

If obesity is always due to one very specific diencephalic deficiency, it follows that the only way to cure it is to correct this deficiency. At first this seemed an utterly hopeless undertaking. The greatest obstacle was that one could hardly hope to correct an inherited trait localized deep inside the brain, and while we did possess a number of drugs whose point of action was believed to be in the diencephalon none of them had the slightest effect on the fat-center. There was not even a pointer showing a direction in which pharmacological research could move to find a drug that had such a specific action. The closest approach wee the appetite-reducing drugs -the amphetamines----- but these cured nothing.

A Curious Observation

Mulling over this depressing situation, I remembered a rather curious observation made many years ago in India. At that time we knew very little about the function of the diencephalon, and my interest centered round the pituitary gland. Proehlich had described eases of extreme obesity and sexual underdevelopment in youths suffering from a new-growth of the anterior pituitary lob, producing what then became known as Froehlich's disease. However, it was very soon discovered that the identical syndrome, though running a less fulminating course, was quite common in patients whose pituitary gland was perfectly normal. These are the so-called "fat boys" with long, slender hands, breasts any flat-chested maiden would be proud to posses, large hips, buttocks and thighs with striation, knock-knees and underdeveloped genitals, often with undescended testicles.

It also became known that in these cases the sex organs could he developed by giving the patients injections of a substance extracted from the urine of pregnant women, it having been shown that when this substance Was injected into sexually immature rats it made them precociously mature. The amount of substance which produced this effect in one rat was called one International Unit, and the purified extract was accordingly called "Human Chorionic Gonadotrophin" whereby chorionic signifies that it is produced in the placenta and gonadotropin that its action is sex gland directed.

The usual way of treating "fat boys" with underdeveloped genitals is to inject several hundred international Units twice a week. Human Chorionic Gonadotrophin which we shall henceforth simply call HCG is expensive and as "fat boys" are fairly common among Indians I tried to establish the smallest effective dose. In the course of this study three interesting things emerged. The first was that when fresh pregnancy-urine from the female ward was given in quantities of about 300 cc. by retention enema, as good results could be obtained as by injecting the pure substance. The second was that small daily doses appeared to be just as effective as much larger ones given twice a week. Thirdly, and that is the observation that concerns us here, when such patients were given small daily doses they seemed to lose their ravenous appetite though rises' neither gained nor lost weight. Strangely enough however, their shape did change. 1 bough they were not restricted in diet, there was a distinct decrease in the circumference of their hips.

Fat on the Move

Remembering this, it occurred to me that the change in shape could only be explained by a movement of fat away from abnormal deposits on the hips, and if that were so there was just a chance that while such fat was in transition it might be available to the body as fuel. This was easy to find out, as in that case fat on the move would be able to replace food. It should then he possible to keep a "fat boy" on a severely restricted diet without a feeling of hunger, in spite of a rapid loss of weight. When I tried this in typical cases of Froehlich's syndrome, I found that as long as such patients were given small daily doses of HCG they could comfortably go about their usual occupations on a diet of only 500 Calories daily and lose an average of about one pound per day. It was also perfectly evident that only Abnormal fat was being consumed, as there were no signs of any depletion of Normal fat. Their skin remained fresh and turgid, and gradually their figures became entirely normal, nor did the daily administration of HCG appear to have any side-effects other than beneficial.

From this point it was a small step to try the same method in all other forms of obesity. It took a few hundred eases to establish beyond reasonable doubt that the mechanism operates in exactly the same way and seemingly without exception in every case of obesity. I found that, though most patients were treated in the out patients department, gross dietary errors rarely occurred on the contrary most patients complained that the two meals of 250 Calories each were more than they could manage, as they continually had a feeling of just having had a large meal.

Pregnancy and Obesity

Once this trail was opened further observations seemed to fall into line, it is, for instance, well known that during pregnancy an. obese woman can very easily lose weight. She can drastically reduce her diet without feeling hunger or discomfort and lose weight without in am nay harming the child in her womb. It is also surprising to what extent a woman can suffer from pregnancy vomiting without coming to any real harm.

Pregnancy is an obese woman's one great chance to reduce her excess weight. 1 hat she so rarely makes use of this opportunity' is due to the erroneous notion, usually fostered by her elder relations, that she now has "two mouths to feed" and must "keep up her strength for the coming event.' All modern obstetricians know that this is nonsense and that the more superfluous fat is lost the less difficult will be tile confinement, though some still hesitate to prescribe a diet sufficiently low in Calories to bring about a drastic reduction.

A woman may gain weight during pregnancy, but she never becomes obese dl tile strict sense of the word. Under the influence of the HCG which circulates in enormous quantities in her body during pregnancy, her diencephalic banking capacity seems to be unlimited, and abnormal fixed deposits are never formed. At confinement she is suddenly deprived of HCG, and her diencephalic fat-center reverts to its normal capacity. It is only then that tile abnormally accumulated fat is locked away in a fixed deposit. From that moment on she is suffering from obesity and is subject to all its consequences.

Pregnancy seems to be the only normal human condition in which the dicncephalic fat banking capacity is unlimited. It is only during pregnancy that fixed fat deposits can be transferred hack into the normal current account and freely drawn upon to make up for any nutritional deficit. During pregnancy every ounce of reserve fat is placed at tile disposal of the growing fetus. Were this not so, an obese woman, whose normal reserves are already depleted, would have the greatest difficulties in bringing her pregnancy to full term. There is considerable evidence to suggest that it is the HCG produced in large quantities in the placenta which brings about this diencephalic change.

Though we may be able to increase the dieneephalic fat banking capacity by injecting HCG, this does not in itself affect the weight, just as transferring monetary funds from a fixed deposit into a current account does not make a man any poorer; to become poorer it is also necessary that he freely spends the money which thus becomes available. In pregnancy the needs of the growing embryo take care of this to some extent, but in the treatment of obesity there is no embryo, and so a very severe dietary restriction must take its place for the duration of treatment.

Only when the fat which is in transit under the effect of HCG is actually consumed can more fat be withdrawn from tile fixed deposits. In pregnancy it would be most undesirable if the fetus were offered ample food only when there is a high influx from the intestinal tract. Ideal nutritional conditions for the fetus can only be achieved when the mother's blood is continually saturated with food, regardless of whether she eats or not, as otherwise a period of starvation might hamper the steady growth of the embryo. It seems that HCG brings about this continual saturation of the blood, which is the reason why obese patients under treatment with HCG never feel hungry in spite of their drastically reduced food intake.

The Nature of Human Chorionic Gonadotroplsin

HCG is never found in the human body except during pregnancy and in those rare cases in which a residue of placental tissue continues to grow in the womb in what is known as a chorionic epithelioma. It is never found in tile male. The human type of chorionic gonadotrophin is found only during the pregnancy of women and the great apes. It is produced in enormous quantities, so that during certain phases of her pregnancy a woman may excrete as much as one million International Units per day in her urine - enough to render a million infantile rats precociously mature. Other mammals make use of a different hormone, which can be extracted from their blood serum but not from their urine. Their placenta differs in this and other respects from that of man and the great apes. This animal choriollic gonadotrophin is much less rapidly broken down in the human body than HCG, and it is also less suitable for the treatment of obesity.

As often happens in medicine, much confusion has been caused by giving HCG its name before its true mode of action was understood. It has been explained that goncidotrophin literally means a sex-gland directed substance or hormone, and this is quite misleading. It dates from the early days when it was first found that HCG is able to render infantile sex glands mature, whereby it was entirely overlooked that it has no stimulating effect whatsoever on normally developed and normally functioning sex-glands. No amount of HCG is ever able to increase a normal sex function it can only improve an abnormal one and in the young hasten the onset of puberty. However, this is no direct effect. HCG acts exclusively at a diencephalic level and there brings about a considerable increase in the functional capacity of all those centers which are working at maximum capacity.

The Real Gonadotrophins

Two hormones known in the female as follicle stimulating hormone (FSH) and corpus luteum stimulating hormone (LSH) are secreted by the anterior lobe of tile pituitary gland. These hormones are real gonadotropilins because they directly govern the function of the ovaries. The anterior pituitary is in turn governed by the diencephalon, and so when there is an ovarian deficiency the diencephalic center concerned is hard put to correct matters by increasing the secretion from the anterior pituitary of FSH or LSH, as the case may be. When sexual deficiency is clinically present, this is a sign that the diencephalic center concerned is unable, in spite of maximal exertion, to cope with the demand for anterior pituitary stimulation. When then the administration of HCG increases the functional capacity of the diencephalon, all demands can be fully satisfied and the sex deficiency is corrected.

That this is the true mechanism underlying the presumed gonadotrophic action of HCG is confirmed by the (act that when the pituitary gland of infantile rats is removed before they are given HCG, the latter has no effect on their sex-glands. HCG cannot therefore have a direct sex gland stimulating action like that of the anterior pituitary gonadotrophins, as FSH and LSH are justly called. The latter are entirely different substances from that which can be extracted from pregnancy urine and which, unfortunately, is called chorionic gonadotiophin. It would be no more clumsy, and certainly far more appropriate, if HCG were henceforth called chorionic dienccphalotrophin.

HCG no Sex Hormone

It cannot he sufficiently emphasized that HCG is not sex- hormone, that its action is identical in men, women, children and in those cases in which the sex-glands no longer function owing to old age or their surgical removal. The only sexual change it can bring about after puberty is an improvement of a pre existing deficiency. But never stimulation beyond the normal in an indirect way via the anterior pituitary HCG regulates menstruation and facilitates conception, but it never virilizes a woman or feminizes a man. It neither makes men grow breasts nor does it interfere with their virility, though where this was deficient it may improve it. It never makes women grow a beard or develop a gruff voice. I have stressed this point only for the sake of my lay readers, because, it is our daily experience that when patients heat the word hormone they immediately jump to the conclusion that this must have something to do with the sex- sphere. They ate not accustomed as we are, to think thyroid insulin, cortisone, adrenalin etc, as hormones.

Importance and Potency of HCG

Owing to the fact that HCG has no direct action on any endocrine gland, its enormous importance in pregnancy has been overlooked and its potency underestimated bough a pregnant woman can produce as much as one million units per day, we find that the injection of only 125 units per day is ample to reduce weight at the rate of roughly one pound per day, even in a colossus weighing 400 pounds, when associated with a 500-Calorie diet.

It is no exaggeration to say that the flooding of the female body with HCG is by far the most spectacular hormonal event in pregnancy. It has an enormous protective importance for mother and child, and I even go so far as to say that no woman, and certainly not an obese one, could carry her pregnancy to term without it.

If I can be forgiven for comparing my fellow-endocrinologists with wicked Godmothers, HCG has certainly been their Cinderella, and I can only romantically hope that its extraordinary effect on Abnormal fat will prove to be its Fairy Godmother.

HCG has been known for over half a century it is the substance which Aschheim and Zondek so brilliantly used to diagnose early pregnancy out of the urine. Apart from that, the only thing it did in the experimental -laboratory was to produce precocious rats, and that was not particularly stimulating to further research at a time when much more thrilling endocrinological discoveries were pouring in from all sides, sweeping, HCG into the stiller back waters.

Complicating Disorders

Some complicating disorders are often associated with obesity, and these we must briefly discuss. The most important associated disorders and the ones in which obesity seems to play a precipitating or at least an aggravating role arc the following the stable type of diabetes, gout, rheumatism and arthritis, high blood pressure and hardening of the arteries, coronary disease and cerebral hemorrhage.

Apart from the fact that they are often-though not necessarily-associated with obesity, these disorders have two things in common. In all of them modern research is becoming more and more inclined to believe that diencephalic regulations play a dominant role in their causation. The other common factor is that they either improve or do not occur during pregnancy. In the latter respect they are joined by many other disorders not necessarily associated with obesity. Such disorders are, for instance, colitis, duodenal or gastric ulcers, certain allergies, psoriasis, loss of hair, brittle fingernails, migraine, etc.

If HCG + diet does in the obese bring about those diencephalic changes which are characteristic of pregnancy, one would expect to see an improvement in all these conditions comparable to that seen in real pregnancy. The administration of HCG does in fact do this in a remarkable way.

Diabetes

In an obese patient suffering from a fairly advanced case of stable diabetes of many years duration in which the blood sugar may range from 3-400 mg%, it is often possible to stop all anti diabetes medication after the first few days of treatment. The blood sugar continues to drop from day to day and often reaches normal values in 2-3 weeks. As in pregnancy, this phenomenon is not observed in the brittle type of diabetes, and as some cases that are predominantly stable may have a small brittle factor in their clinical makeup, all obese diabetics have to be kept under a very careful and expert watch.

A brittle diabetes is primarily due to the inability of the pancreas to produce sufficient insulin, while in the stable type diencephalic regulations seem to be of greater importance. That is possibly the reason why the stable form responds so well to the HCG method of treating obesity, whereas the brittle type does not. Obese patients are generally suffering from the stable type, but a stable type may gradually change into a brittle one, which is usually associated with a loss of weight. Thus when an obese diabetic finds that he is losing weight without diet or treatment, he should at once have his diabetes expertly attended to. There is some evidence to suggest that the change from stable to brittle is more liable to occur in patients who are taking insulin for their stable diabetes.

Rheumatism

All rheumatic pains, even those associated with demonstrable bony lesions, improve subjectively within a few days of treatment, and often require neither cortisone nor salicylates. Again this is a well known phenomenon in pregnancy, and while under treatment with HCG + diet the effect is no less dramatic. As it does not alter pregnancy, the pain of deformed joints returns after treatment, but smaller doses of pain-relieving drugs seem able to control it satisfactorily after weight reduction. In any case, the HCG method makes it possible in obese arthritic patients to interrupt prolonged cortisone treatment without a recurrence of pain. This in itself is most welcome, but there is the added advantage that the treatment stimulates the secretion of ACTH in a physiological manner and that this regenerates the adrenal cortex, which is apt to suffer under prolonged cortisone treatment.

Cholesterol

The exact extent to which the blood cholesterol is involved in hardening of the arteries, high blood pressure and coronary disease is not as yet known, but it is now widely admitted that the blood cholesterol level is governed by diencephalic mechanisms. The behavior of circulating cholesterol is therefore of particular interest during the treatment of obesity with HCG. Cholesterol circulates in two forms, which we call free and esterified. Normally these fractions are present in a proportion of about 25% free to 75gb esterified cholesterol, and it is the latter fraction which damages the walls of the arteries. In pregnancy this proportion is reversed and it may be taken for granted that arteriosclerosis never gets worse during pregnancy for this very reason.

To my knowledge, the only other condition in which the proportion of free to esterified cholesterol is reversed is during the treatment of obesity with HCG+ diet, when exactly the same phenomenon takes place. This seems an important indication of how closely a patient under HCG treatment resembles a pregnant woman in diencephalic behavior.

When the total amount of circulating cholesterol is normal before treatment, this absolute amount is neither significantly increased nor decreased. But when an obese patient with an abnormally high cholesterol and already showing signs of arteriosclerosis is treated with HCG, his blood pressure drops and his coronary circulation seems to improve, and yet his total blood cholesterol may soar to heights never before reached.

At first this greatly alarmed us. But when we saw that the patients came to no harm even if treatment was continued and we found in follow-up examinations undertaken some months after treatment was continued and we found in follow-up examinations undertaken some months before treatment. As the increase is mostly in the form of the not dangerous form of the free cholesterol, we gradually came to welcome the phenomenon. Today we believe that the rise is entirely due to the liberation of recent cholesterol deposits that have not yet undergone calcification in the arterial wall and therefore highly beneficial.

Gout

An identical behavior is found in the blood uric acid level of patient suffering from gout. Predictably such patients get an acute and often severe attack after the first few days of HCG treatment but then remain entirely free of pain, in spite of the fact that their blood uric acid often shows a marked increase which may persist for several months after treatment. Those patients who have regained their normal weight remain free of symptoms regardless of what they eat, while those that require a second course of treatment get another attack of gout as soon as the second course is initiated. We do not yet know what dioncephalic mechanisms arc involved in gout; possibly emotional factors play a role, and it is worth remembering that the disease clues not occur in women of childbearing age. We now give 2 tablets daily of ZYLORIC to all patients who give a history of gout and have a high blood uric acid level. In this way we can completely avoid attacks during treatment.

Blood Pressure

Patients, who have brought themselves to the brink of malnutrition by exaggerated dieting, laxatives etc, often have an abnormally low blood pressure. In these cases the blood pressure rises to normal values at the beginning of treatment and then very gradually drops, as it always does in patients with a normal blood pressure. Normal values are always regained a few days after the treatment is over. Of this lowering of the blood pressure during treatment the patients are not aware. When the blood pressure is abnormally high, and provided there are no detectable renal lesions, the pressure drops, as it usually does in pregnancy. The drop is often very rapid, so rapid in fact that sometimes advisable to slow down the process with pressure sustaining medication until the circulation has had a few days time to adjust itself the new situation. On the other hand, among the thousands cases treated we have never seen any untoward incident which could be attributed to the rather sudden drop in high blood pressure.

When a woman suffering from high blood pressure becomes pregnant her blood pressure very soon drops, but after her confinement it may gradually rise back to its former level. Similarly, a high blood pressure present before HCG treatment tends to rise again after the treatment is over, though this is not always the case. But the former high levels are rarely reached, and we have gathered the impression that such relapses respond better to orthodox drugs such as Reserpine than before treatment.

Peptic Ulcers

In our cases of obesity with gastric or duodenal ulcers we have noticed a surprising subjective improvement in spite of a diet which would generally be considered most inappropriate for an ulcer patient. Here, too, there is a similarity with pregnancy, in which peptic ulcers hardly ever occur. However we have seen two cases with a previous history of several hemorrhages in which a bleeding occurred within 2 weeks of the end of treatment.

Psoriasis, Fingernails, Hair Varicose Ulcers

As in pregnancy, psoriasis greatly improves during treatment but may relapse when the treatment is over. Most patients spontaneously report a marked improvement in the condition of brittle fingernails. The loss of hair not infrequently associated with obesity is temporarily arrested, though in very rare cases an increased loss of hair has been reported. I remember a case in which a patient developed a patchy baldness - so called alopecia areata - after a severe emotional shock, just before she was about to start an HCG treatment. Our dermatologist diagnosed the case as a particularly severe one, predicting that all the hair would be lost. He counseled against the reducing treatment, but in view of my previous experience and as the patient was very anxious not to postpone reducing, I discussed the matter with the dermatologist and it was agreed that, having fully acquainted the patient with the situation, the treatment should be started. During the treatment, which lasted four weeks, the further development of the bald patches was almost, if not quite, arrested; however, within a week of having finished the course of HCG, all the remaining hair fell out as predicted by the dermatologist. The interesting point is that the treatment was able to postpone this result but not to prevent it. The patient has now grown a new shock of hair of which she is justly proud.

In obese patients with large varicose ulcers we were surprised to find that these ulcers heal rapidly under treatment with HCG. We have since treated non obese patients suffering from varicose ulcers with daily injections of HCG on normal diet with equally good results.

The "Pregnant" Male

When a male patient hears that he is about to be put into a condition which in some respects resembles pregnancy, he is usually shocked and horrified. The physician must therefore carefully explain that this does not mean that he will be feminized and that HCG in no way interferes with his sex. He must be made to understand that in the interest of the propagation of the species nature provides for a perfect functioning of the regulatory head quarters in the diencephalun during pregnancy and that we are merely using this natural safeguard as a means of correcting the dicncephalic disorder which is responsible for his overweight.

Technique

Warnings

I must warn the lay reader that what follows is mainly for the treating physician and most certainly not a do it-yourself primer. Many of the expressions used mean something entirely different to a qualified doctor than that which their common use implies, and only a physician can correctly interpret the symptoms which may arise during treatment. Any patient who thinks he can reduce by taking a few "shots" and eating less is not only sure to be disappointed but may be heading for serious trouble. The benefit the patient can derive from reading this part of the book is a fuller realization of how very important it is for him to follow to the letter his physician's instructions.

In treating obesity with the HCG + diet method we are handling what is perhaps the most complex organ in the human body. The diencephalon's functional equilibrium is delicately poised, so that whatever happens in one part has repercussions in others. In obesity this balance is out of kilter and can only be restored if the technique I am about to describe is followed implicitly. Even seemingly insignificant deviations, particularly those that at first sight seem to be an improvement, are very liable to produce most disappointing results and even annul the effect completely. For instance, if the diet is increased from 500 to 600 or 700 Calories, the loss of weight is quite unsatisfactory. If the daily dose of HCG is raised to 200 or more units daily its action often appears to be reversed, possibly because larger doses evoke diencephalic counter-regulations. On the other hand, the diencephalon is an extremely robust organ in spite of its unbelievable intricacy. From an evolutionary point of view it is one of the oldest organs in our body and its evolutionary history dates back more than 500 million years. 'This has tendered it extraordinarily adapt able to all natural exigencies, and that is one of the main reasons why the human species was able to evolve what its evolution did not prepare it for were the conditions to which human culture and civilization expose it.

History Taking

When a patient first presents himself for treatment, we take a general history and note the time when the first signs of overweight were observed. We try to establish the highest weight the patient has ever had in his life (obviously excluding pregnancy), when this was and what measures have hitherto been taken in an effort to reduce.

It has been our experience that those patients who have been taking thyroid preparations for long periods have a slightly lower average loss of weight under treatment with HCG than those who have never taken thyroid. This is even so in those patients who have been taking thyroid because they had an abnormally low basal metabolic rate. In many of these cases the low BMR is not due to any intrinsic deficiency of the thyroid gland, but rather to a lack of diencephalic stimulation of the thyroid gland via the anterior pituitary lobe. We never allow thyroid to be taken during treatment, and yet a BMR which was very low before treatment is usually found to be normal after a week or two of HCG + diet. Needless to say, this does not apply to those cases in which a thyroid deficiency has been produced by the surgical removal of a part of an overactive gland. It is also most important to ascertain whether the patient has taken diuretics (water eliminating pills) as this also decreases the weight loss under the HCG regimen.

Returning to our procedure, we next ask the patient a few questions to which he is held to reply simply with "yes" or "no". These questions are: Do you suffer from headaches? rheumatic pains? menstrual disorders? constipation? breathlessness or exertion? swollen ankles? Do you consider yourself greedy? Do you feel the need to eat snacks between meals? The patient then strips and is weighed and measured. The normal weight for his height, age, skeletal and muscular build is established from tables of statistical averages, whereby in women it is often necessary to make an allowance for particularly large and heavy breasts. The degree of overweight is then calculated, and from this the duration of treatment can be roughly assessed on the basis of an average loss of weight of a little less than a pound say 300-400 grams-per injection and day. It is a particularly interesting feature of the HCG treatment that in reasonably cooperative patients this figure is remarkably constant, regardless of sex, age and degree of overweight.

The Duration of Treatment

Patients who need to lose 15 pounds (7 kg.) or less require 26 days treatment with 23 daily injections. The extra three days are needed because all patients must continue the 500- Calorie diet for three days after the last injection. This is a very essential part of the treatment, because if they start eating normally as long as there is even a trace of HCG in their body they put on weight alarmingly at the end of the treatment. After three days when all the HCG has been eliminated this does not happen, because the blood is then no longer saturated with food and can thus accommodate an extra influx from the intestines without increasing its volume by retaining water.

We never give a treatment lasting less than 26 days, even in patients needing to lose only 5 pounds. It seems that even in the mildest cases of obesity the diencephalon requires about three weeks rest from the maximal exertion to which it has been previously subjected in order to regain fully its Normal fat banking capacity. Clinically this expresses itself -in the fact that when in these mild cases treatment is stopped as soon as the weight is normal, which may be achieved in a week, it is much more easily regained than after a full course of 23 injections.

As soon as such patients have lost all their abnormal superfluous fat, they at once begin to feel ravenously hungry in she of continued injections. This is because HCG only puts Abnormal fat into circulation and cannot, in the doses used, liberate Normal fat deposits; indeed, it seems to prevent their consumption. As soon as their statistically normal weight is reached, these patients are put on 800-1000 calories for the rest of the treatment. The diet is arranged in such a way that the weight remains perfectly stationary and is thus continued for three days after the 23rd injection. Only then are the patients free to eat anything they please except sugar and starches for the next three weeks.

Such early cases are common among actresses, models, mannequins and persons who are tired of obesity, having seen its ravages in other members of their family. Film actresses frequently explain that they must weigh less than normal. With this request we flatly refuse to comply, first, because we undertake to cure a disorder, not to create a new one, and second, because it is in the nature of the HCG method that it is self limiting. It becomes completely ineffective as soon as all Abnormal fat is consumed. Actresses with a slight tendency to obesity, having tried all manner of reducing methods, invariably come to the conclusion that their figure is satisfactory only when they are underweight, simply because none of these methods remove their superfluous fat deposits. When they see that under HCG their figure improves out of all proportion to the amount of weight lost, they are nearly always content to remain within their normal weight-range.

When a patient has more than 15 pounds to lose the treatment takes longer but the maximum we give in a single course is 40 injections, nor do we as a rule allow patients to lose more than 34 lbs. (15 Kg.) at a time. The treatment is stopped when either 34 lbs. have been lost or 40 injections have been given. The only exception we make is in the case of grotesquely obese patients who may be allowed to lose an additional 5-6 lbs. if this occurs before the 40 injections are up.

Immunity to HCG

The reason for limiting a course to 40 injections is that by then some patients may begin to show signs of HCG immunity. Though this phenomenon is well known, we cannot as yet define the underlying mechanism. Maybe after a certain length of time the body learns to break down and eliminate HCG very rapidly, or possibly prolonged treatment leads to some sort of counter-regulation which annuls the dencepbahic effect.

After 40 daily injections it takes about six weeks before this so called immunity is lost and HCG again becomes fully effective. Usually after about 40 injections patients may feel the onset of immunity as hunger which was previously absent. In those comparatively rare cases in which signs of immunity develop before the full course of 40 injections has been completed-say at the 35th injection- treatment must he stopped at once, because if it is continued the patients begin to look weary and drawn, feel weak and hungry and any further loss of weight achieved is then always at the expense of Normal fat. This is not only undesirable, but Normal fat is also instantly regained as soon as the patient is returned to a free diet.

Patients who need only 23 injections may be injected daily, including Sundays, as they never develop immunity. In those that take 40 injections the onset of immunity can be delayed if they are given only six injections a week, leaving out Sundays or any other day they choose, provided that it is always the same day. On the days on which they do not receive the injections they usually feel a slight sensation of hunger. At first we thought that this might be purely psychological, but we found that when normal saline is injected without the patient's knowledge the same phenomenon occurs.

Menstruation

During menstruation no injections are given, but the diet is continued and causes no hardship; yet as soon as the menstruation is over, the patients become extremely hungry unless the injections are resumed at once. It is very impressive to see the suffering of a woman who has continued her diet for a day or two beyond the end of the period without coming for her injection and then to hear the next day that all hunger ceased within a few hours after the injection and to see her once again content, florid and cheerful. While on the question of menstruation it must he added that in teenage girls the period may in some rare cases he delayed and exceptionally stop altogether. If then later this is artificially induced some weight may be regained.

Further Courses

Patients requiring losing more than 34 lbs. must have a second or even more courses. A second course can be started after an interval of not less than six weeks, though the pause can be more than six weeks. When a third, fourth or even fifth course is necessary, the interval between courses should be made progressively longer. Between a second and third course eight weeks should elapse, between a third and fourth course twelve weeks, between a fourth and fifth course twenty weeks and between a fifth and sixth course six months. In this way it is possible to bring about a weight reduction of 100 lbs. and more if required without the least hardship to the patient.

In general, men do slightly better than women and often reach a somewhat higher average daily loss. Very advanced cases do a little better than early ones, but it is a remarkable fact that this difference is only just statistically significant.

Conditions that Must be Accepted Before Treatment

On the basis of these data the probable duration of treatment can he calculated with considerable accuracy and this is explained to the patient. It is made clear to him that during the course of treatment he must attend the clinic daily to be weighed, injected and generally checked. All patients that live in Rome or have resident friends or relations with whom they can stay are treated as out-patients, but patients coming from abroad must stay in the hospital, as no hotel or restaurant can be relied upon to prepare the diet with sufficient accuracy. These patients have their meals, sleep and attend the clinic in the hospital, but are otherwise free to spend their time as they please in the city and its surroundings sightseeing bathing or theater-going. It is also made clear that between courses the patient gets no treatment and is free to eat anything he pleases except starches and sugar during the first 3 weeks. It is impressed upon him that he will have to follow the prescribed diet to the letter and that after the first three days this will cost him no effort, as he will feel no hunger and may indeed have difficulty in getting down the 500 Calories which he will be given. If these conditions are not acceptable the case is refused, as any compromise or half measure is bound to prove utterly disappointing to patient and physician alike and is a waste of time and energy.

Though a patient can only consider himself really cured when he has been reduced to his statistically normal weight, we do not insist that he commit himself to that extent. Even a partial loss of overweight is highly beneficial, and it is our experience that once a patient has completed a first course he is so enthusiastic about the ease with which the-to him surprising-results are achieved that he almost invariably comes back for more. There certainly can be no doubt that in my clinic more time is spent on damping over-enthusiasm than on insisting that the rules of the treatment be observed.

Examining the patient

Only when agreement is reached on the points so far discussed do we proceed with the examination of the patient. A note is made of the size of the first upper incisor, of a pad of fat on the nape of the neck, at the axilla and on the inside of the knees. The presence of striation, a suprapubic fold, a thoracic fold, angulation of elbow and knee joint, breast-development in men and women, edema of the ankles and the state of genital development in the male are noted.

Wherever this seems indicated we X-ray the sella turcica, as the bony capsule which contains the pituitary gland is called, measure the basal metabolic rate, X-ray the chest and take an electrocardiogram. We do a blood-count and a sedimentation rate and estimate uric acid, cholesterol, iodine and sugar in the fasting blood.

Gain Before Loss

Patients whose general condition is low, owing to excessive previous dieting, must eat to capacity for about one week before starting treatment, regardless of how much weight they may gain in the process. One cannot keep a patient comfortably on 500 Calories unless his Normal fat reserves are reasonably well stocked. It is for this reason also that every case, even those that are actually gaining must eat to capacity of the most fattening food they can get down until they have had then third injection. It is a fundamental mistake to put a patient on 500 Calories as soon as the injections are started, as it seems to take about three injections before abnormally deposited fat begins to circulate and thus become available.

We distinguish between the first three injections, which we call 'non-effective' as far as the loss of weight is concerned, and the subsequent injections given while the patient is dieting, which we call "effective". The average loss of weight is calculated on the number of effective injections and from the weight reached on the day of the third injections which may he well above what it was two days earlier when the first injection as given. Most patients who have been struggling with diets for years and know how rapidly they gain if they let themselves go are very hard to convince of the absolute necessity of gorging for at least two days, and yet this must he insisted upon categorically if the further course of treatment is to run smoothly. Those patients who have to be put on forced feeding for a week before starting the injections usually gain weight rapidly- four to six pounds in 24 hours is not unusual-but after a day or two this rapid gain generally levels off. In any case the whole gain is usually lost in the first 48 hours of dieting. It is necessary to proceed in this manner because the gain re-stocks the depleted normal reserves, whereas the Subsequent loss is from the abnormal deposits only. Patients in a satisfactory general condition and those who have not just previously restricted their diet start forced feeding on the day of the first injection. Some patents say that they can no longer overeat because their stomach has shrunk after years of restrictions. While we know that no stomach ever shrinks, we compromise by insisting that they eat frequently of highly concentrated foods such as milk chocolate, pastries with whipped cream sugar, fried meats particularly pork, eggs and bacon, mayonnaise, bread with thick butter and jam, etc. The time and trouble spent on pressing this point upon incredulous or reluctant patients is always amply rewarded afterwards by the complete absence of those difficulties which patients who have disregarded these instructions are liable to experience.

During the two days of forced feeding from the first to the third injection - many patients are surprised that contrary to their previous experience they do not gain weight and some even lose. The explanation is that in these cases there is a compensatory flow of urine, which drains excessive water from the body. To some extent this seems to be a direct action of HCG, but it may also be due to a higher protein intake, as we know that a protein-deficient diet makes the body retain water.

Starting Treatment

In menstruating women the best time to start treatment is immediately after a period. Treatment may also be started later, but it is advisable to have at least ten days in hand before the onset of the next period. Similarly, the end of a course of onset should never be made to coincide with menstruation. If things should happen to work out that way, it is better to give the last injection three days before the expected date of the menses so that a normal diet can he resumed at onset. Alternatively, at least three injections should be given after the period, followed by the usual three days of dieting This rule need not be observed in such patients who have reached their normal weight before the end of treatment and are already on a higher caloric diet.

Patients who require more than the minimum of 23 injections and who therefore skip one day a week in order to postpone immunity to HCG cannot have their third injections on the day before the interval. Thus if it is decided to skip Sundays, the treatment can be started on any day of the week except Thursdays. Supposing they start on Thursday, they will have their third injection on Saturday, which is also the day on which they start their 500 Calorie diet. They would then base no injection on the second day of dieting, this exposes them to an unnecessary hardship, as without the injection they will feel particularly hungry. Of course, the difficulty can be overcome by exceptionally injecting them on the first Sunday. If this day falls between the first and second or between the second and third injection, we usually prefer to give the patient the extra day of forced feeding, which the majority rapturously enjoy.

The Diet

The 500 calorie diet is explained on the day of the second injection to those patients who will be preparing their own food, and it is most important that the person who will actually cook is present - the wife, the mother or the cook, as the case may be. Here in Italy patients are given the following diet sheet.

Breakfast :	Tea or coffee in any quantity without sugar. Only one tablespoonful of milk allowed in 24 hours. Saccharin or other sweeteners may be used. (*Written before studies linking Saccharin to Cancer and the availability of Stevia – we recommend using Stevia instead*)

202

Lunch:

1. 100 grams of veal, beef, chicken breast, fresh white fish, lobster, crab, or shrimp. All visible fat must be carefully removed before cooking, and the meat must be weighed raw. It must be boiled or grilled without additional fat. Salmon, eel, tuna, herring, dried or pickled fish are not allowed. The chicken must be removed from the bird.

2. One type of vegetable only to be chosen from the following: spinach, chard, chicory, beet-greens, green salad, tomatoes, celery, fennel, onions, red radishes, cucumbers, asparagus, cabbage.

3. One breadstick (grissino) or one Melba toast.

4. An apple or a handful of strawberries or one-half grapefruit.

Dinner :   The same four choices as lunch.

The juice of one lemon daily is allowed for all purposes. Salt, pepper, vinegar, mustard powder, garlic, sweet basil, parsley, thyme, marjoram, etc., may be used for seasoning, but no oil, butter or dressing.

Tea, coffee, plain water, mineral water are the only drinks allowed, but they may be taken in any quantity and at all times.

In fact the patient should drink about 2 liters of these fluids per day. Many patients are afraid to drink so much because they fear that this may make them retain more water. This is a wrong notion as the body is more inclined to store water when the intake falls below its normal requirements.

The fruit or the breadstick may be eaten between meals instead of with lunch or dinner, but not more than four items listed for lunch and dinner may be eaten at one meal.

No medicines or cosmetics other than lipstick eyebrow pencil and powder may he used without special permission

Every item in the list is gone over carefully, continually stressing the point that no variations other than those listed may be introduced. All things not listed are forbidden, and the patient is assured that nothing permissible has been left out. The 100 grams of meat must he scrupulously weighed raw after all visible fat has been removed to do this accurately the patient must have a letter-scale, as kitchen scales are not sufficiently accurate and the butcher should certainly not be relied upon. Those not uncommon patients, who feel that even so little food is too much for them, can omit anything they wish.

There is no objection to breaking up the two meals. For instance: having a breadstick and an apple for breakfast or an orange before going to bed, provided they are deducted from the regular meals. The whole daily ration of two breadsticks or two fruits may not be eaten at the same time, nor can any item saved from the previous day be added on the following day. In the beginning patients are advised to check every meal again their diet sheet before starting to eat and not to rely on their memory. It is also worth pointing out that any attempt to observe this diet without HCG will lead to trouble in two to three days. We have had cases in which patients have proudly flaunted their dieting powers in front of their friends without mentioning the fact that they are also receiving treatment with HCG. They let their friends try the same diet, and when this proves to be a failure - as it necessarily must - the patient starts raking in unmerited kudos for superhuman willpower. It should also be mentioned that two small apples weighing as much as one large one never the less have a higher caloric value and are therefore not allowed though there is no restriction on the size of one apple. Some people do not realize that a tangerine is not an orange and that thicken breast does not mean the breast of any other fowl, nor does it mean a wing or drumstick.

The most tiresome patients are those who start counting Calories and then come up with all manner of ingenious variations which they compile from their little books. When one has spent years of weary research trying to make a diet as attractive as possible without jeopardizing the loss of weight, culinary geniuses who are out to improve their unhappy lot are hard to take.

Making up the Calories

The diet used in conjunction with HCG must not exceed 500 Calories per day, and the way these Calories are made up is of utmost importance. For instance, if a patient drops the apple and eats an extra breadstick instead, he will not be getting more Calories but he will not lose weight. There are a number of foods, particularly fruits and vegetables, which have the same or even lower caloric values than those listed as permissible, and yet we find that they interfere with the regular loss of weight under HCG, presumably owing to the nature of their composition. Pimiento peppers, okra, artichokes and pears are examples of this.

While this diet works satisfactorily in Italy, certain modifications have to be made in other countries. For instance, American beef has almost double the caloric value of South Italian beef, which is not marbled with fat. This marbling is impossible to remove. In America, therefore, low-grade veal should be used for one meal and fish (excluding all those species such as herring, mackerel, tuna, salmon, eel, etc., which have a high fat content, and all dried, smoked or pickled fish), chicken breast, lobster, crawfish, pawns shrimps, crabmeat or kidneys for the other meal. Where the Italian breadsticks, the so-called grissini, are not available one Melba toast may be used instead, though they are psychologically less satisfying. A Melba toast has about the same weight as the very porous grissini which is much more to look at and to chew.

In many countries specially prepared unsweetened and low Calorie foods are freely available, and some of these can be tentatively used. When local conditions or the feeding habits of the population make changes necessary it must be borne in mind that the total daily intake must not exceed 500 Calories if the best possible results are to be obtained, that the daily ration should contain 200 grams of fat-free protein and a very small amount of starch.

Just as the daily dose of HCG is the same in all cases, so the same diet proves to be satisfactory for a small elderly lady of leisure or a hard working muscular giant. Under the effect of HCG the obese body is always able to obtain all the Calories it needs from the Abnormal fat deposits, regardless of whether it uses up 1500 or 4000 per day. It must be made very clear to the patient that he is living to a far greater extent on the fat which he is losing than on what he eats.

Many patients ask why eggs are not allowed. The contents of two good sized eggs are roughly equivalent to 100 grams of meat, but fortunately the yolk contains a large amount of fat, which is undesirable. Very occasionally we allow egg - boiled, poached or raw - to patients who develop an aversion to meat, but in this case they must add the white of three eggs to the one they eat whole. In countries where cottage cheese made from skimmed milk is available 100 grams may occasionally be used instead of the meat, but no other cheeses are allowed.

Vegetarians

Strict vegetarians such as orthodox Hindus present a special problem, because milk and curds are the only animal protein they will eat. To supply them with sufficient protein of animal origin they must drink 500 cc. of skimmed milk per day, though part of this ration can be taken as curds. As far as fruit, vegetables and starch are concerned, their diet is the same as that of non- vegetarians; they cannot be allowed their usual intake of vegetable proteins from leguminous plants such as beans or from wheat or nuts, nor can they have their customary rice. In spite of these severe restrictions, their average loss is about half that of non vegetarians, presumably owing to the sugar content of the milk.

Faulty Dieting

Few patients will take one's word for it that the slightest deviation from the diet has under HCG disastrous results as far as the weight is concerned. This extreme sensitivity has the advantage that the smallest error is immediately detectable at the daily weighing but most patients have to make the experience before they will believe it.

Persons in high official positions such as embassy personnel, politicians, senior executives, etc., who are obliged to attend social functions to which they cannot bring their meager meal must be told beforehand that an official dinner will cost them the loss of about three days treatment, however careful they are and in spite of a friendly and would-be cooperative host. 'We generally advise them to avoid all-round embarrassment, the almost inevitable turn of conversation to their weight problem and the outpouring of lay counsel from their table partners by not letting it be known that they are under treatment. They should take dainty servings of everything, bide what they can under the cutlery and book the gain which may take three days to get rid of as one of the sacrifices which their profession entails. Allowing three days for their correction such incidents do not jeopardize the treatment, provided they do not occur all too frequently in which case treatment should be postponed to a socially more peaceful season.

Vitamins and Anemia

Sooner or later most patients express a fear that they may be running out of vitamins or that the restricted diet may make them anemic. On this score the physician can confidently relieve their apprehension by explaining that every time they lose a pound of fatty tissue, which they do almost daily, only the actual fat is burned up; all the vitamins, the proteins the blood and the minerals which this tissue contains in abundance are fed back into the body Actually, a low blood count not due to any serious disorder of the blood forming tissues improves during treatment, and we have never encountered a significant protein deficiency nor signs of a lack of vitamins in patients who are dieting regularly.

The First Days of Treatment

On the day of the third injection it is almost routine to hear two remarks. One is: "You know, Doctor, I'm sure it's only psychological, but I already feel quite different". So common is this remark, even from very skeptical patients that we hesitate to accept the psychological interpretation. The other typical remark is: "Now that I have been allowed to eat anything I want, I can't get it down. Since yesterday I feel like a stuffed pig. Food just doesn't seem to interest me anymore, and I am longing to get on with your diet". Many patients notice that they are passing more urine and that the swelling in their ankles is less even before they start dieting. On the day of the fourth injection most patients declare that they are feeling fine. They have usually lost two pounds or more, some say they feel a bit empty but hasten to explain that this does not amount to hunger. Some complain of a mild headache of which they have been forewarned and for which they have been given permission to take aspirin. During the second and third day of dieting - that is, the fifth and sixth injection- these minor complaints improve while the weight continues to drop at about double the usually overall average of almost one pound per day, so that a moderately severe case may by the fourth day of dieting have lost as much as 8- 10 lbs. It is usually at this point that a difference appears between those patients who have literally eaten to capacity during the first two days of treatment and those who have not. The former feel remarkably well; they have no hunger, nor do they feel tempted when others eat normally at the same table. They feel lighter, more clear-headed and notice a desire to move quite contrary to their previous lethargy. Those who have disregarded the advice to eat to capacity continue to have minor discomforts and do not have the same euphoric sense of self-being until about a week later. It seems that their Normal fat reserves require that much more time before they are fully stocked.

Fluctuations in Weight Loss

After the fourth or fifth day of dieting the daily loss of weight begins to decrease to one pound or somewhat less per clay, and there is a smaller urinary output. Men often continue to lose regularly at that rate, but women are more irregular in spite of faultless dieting. There may be no drop at all for two or three days and then a sudden loss which reestab1ishes the normal average. These fluctuations are entirely due to variations in the retention and elimination of water, which are more marked in women than in men.

The weight registered by the scale is determined by two processes not necessarily synchronized under the influence of HCG fat is being extracted from the cells, in which it is stored in the fatty tissue. When these cells are empty and therefore serve o purpose the body breaks down the cellular structure and absorbs it, but breaking up of useless cells, connective tissue, blood vessels, etc., may lag behind the process of fat-extraction. When this happens the body appears to replace some of the extracted fat with water which is retained for this purpose. As water is heavier than fat the scales may show no loss of weight, although sufficient fat has actually been consumed to make up for the deficit in the 500-Calorie diet. When then such tissue is finally broken down, the water is liberated and there is a sudden flood of urine and a marked loss of weight. This simple interpretation of what is really an extremely complex mechanism is the one we give those patients who want to know why it is that on certain days they do not lose, though they have committed no dietary error.

Patients who have previously regularly used diuretics as a method of reducing lose fat during the first two or three weeks of treatment which shows in their measurements, but the scale may show little or no loss because they are replacing the normal water content of their body which has been dehydrated. Diuretics should never be used for reducing.

Interruptions of Weight Loss

We distinguish four types of interruption in the regular daily loss. The first is the one that has already been mentioned in which the weight stays stationary for a day or two, and this occurs, particularly towards the end of a course, in almost every case.

The Plateau

The second type of interruption we call a "plateau". A plateau lasts 4-6 days and frequently occurs during the second half of a full course, particularly in patients that have been doing well and whose overall average of nearly a pound per effective injection has been maintained. Those who are losing more than the average all have a plateau sooner or later. A plateau always corrects, itself, but many patients who have become accustomed to a regular daily loss get unnecessarily worried and begin to bet. No amount of explanation convinces them that a plateau does not mean that they are no longer responding normally to treatment.

In such cases we consider it permissible, for purely psychological reasons, to break up the plateau. This can be done in two ways. One is a so-called "apple day". An apple-day begins at lunch and continues until just before lunch of the following day. The patients are given six large apples and are told to eat one whenever they feel the desire though six apples is the maximum allowed. During an apple-day no other food or liquids except plain water are allowed and of water they may only drink just enough to quench an uncomfortable thirst if eating an apple still leaves them thirsty. Most patients feel no need for water and are quite happy with their six apples. Needless to say, an apple-day may never be given on the day on which there is no injection. The apple-day produces a gratifying loss of weight on the following day, chiefly due to the elimination of water. This water is not regained when the patients resume their normal 500- Calorie diet at lunch, and on the following days they continue to lose weight satisfactorily.

The other way to break up a plateau is by giving a non- mercurial diuretic for one day. This is simpler for the patient but we prefer the apple-day as we sometimes find that though the diuretic is very effective on the following day it may take two to three days before the normal daily reduction is resumed, throwing the patient into a new fit of despair. It is useless to give either an apple-day or a diuretic unless the weight has been stationary for at least four days without any dietary error having been committed.

Reaching a Former Level
The third type of interruption in the regular loss of weight may last much longer-ten days to two weeks. Fortunately, it is rare and only occurs in very advanced cases, and then hardly ever during the first course of treatment. It is seen only in those patients who during some period of their lives have maintained a certain fixed degree of obesity for ten years or more and have then at some time rapidly increased beyond that weight. When then in the course of treatment the former level is reached, it may take two weeks of no loss, in spite of HCG and diet, before further reduction is normally resumed.

Menstrual Interruption
The fourth type of interruption is the one which often occurs a few days before and during the menstrual period and in some women at the time of ovulation. It must also be mentioned that when a woman becomes pregnant during treatment - and this is by no means uncommon - she at once ceases to lose weight. An unexplained arrest

of reduction has on several occasions raised our suspicion before the first period was missed. If in such eases menstruation is delayed, we stop injecting and do a precipitation test five days later. No pregnancy test should be carried out earlier than five days after the last injection, as otherwise the HCG may give a false positive result.

Oral contraceptives may be used during treatment.

Dietary Errors

Any interruption of the normal loss of weight which does not fit perfectly into one of those categories is always due to some possibly very minor dietary error. Similarly, any gain of more than 100 grams is invariably the result of some transgression or mistake, unless it happens on or about the day of ovulation or during the three days preceding the onset of menstruation, in which case it is ignored. In all other cases the reason for the gain must be established at once.

The patient who frankly admits that he has stepped out of his regimen when told that something has gone wrong is no problem. He is always surprised at being found out, because unless he has seen this himself he will not believe that a salted almond, a couple of potato chips, a glass of tomato juice or an extra orange will bring about a definite increase in his weight on the following day.
Very often he wants to know why extra food weighing one ounce should increase his by six ounces. We explain this in the following way: Under the influence of HCG the blood is saturated with food and the blood volume has adapted itself so that it can only just accommodate the 500 Calories which come in from the intestinal tract in the course of the day. Any additional income, however little this may be, cannot be accommodated and the blood is therefore forced to increase its volume sufficiently to hold the extra food, which it can only do in a very diluted form. Thus it is not the weight of what is eaten that plays the determining role but rather the amount of water which the body must retain to accommodate this food.

This can be illustrated by mentioning the case of salt. In order to hold one teaspoonful of salt the body requires one liter of water, as it cannot accommodate salt in any higher concentration. Thus, if a person eats one teaspoonful of salt his weight will go up by more than two pounds as soon as this salt is absorbed from his intestine. To this explanation many patients reply: Well, if I put on that much every time I eat a little extra, how can I hold my weight after the treatment It must therefore be made clear that this only happens as long as they are under HCG. When treat melt is over, the blood is no longer saturated and can easily accommodate extra food without having to increase its volume. Here again the professional reader will he aware that this interpretation is a simplification of an extremely intricate physiological process which actually accounts for the phenomenon.

Salt and Reducing

While we are on the subject of salt, I can take this opportunity to explain that we make no restriction in the use of salt and insist that the patients drink large quantities of water throughout the treatment. We are out to reduce Abnormal fat and are not in the least interested in such illusory weight losses as can be achieved by depriving the body of salt and by desiccating it. Though we allow the free use of salt, the daily amount taken should be roughly the same, as a sudden increase will of course be followed by a corresponding increase in weight as shown by the scale. An increase in the intake of salt is one of the most common causes for an increase in weight from one day to the next. Such an increase can be ignored, provided it is accounted for, it in no way influences the regular loss of fat.

Water

Patients are usually hard to convince that the amount of water they retain has nothing to do with the amount of water they drink. When the body is forced to retain water, it will do this at all costs. If the fluid intake is insufficient to provide all the water required, the body withholds water from the kidneys and the urine becomes scanty and highly concentrated, imposing a certain strain on the kidneys. If that is insufficient, excessive water will be with-drawn from the intestinal tract, with the result that the feces become hard and dry. On the other hand if a patient drinks more than his body requires, the surplus is promptly and easily eliminated. Trying to prevent the body from retaining water by drinking less is therefore not only futile but even harmful.

Constipation

An excess of water keeps the feces soft, and that is very important in the obese, who commonly suffer from Constipation and a spastic colon. While a patient is under treatment we never permit the use of any kind of laxative taken by mouth. We explain that owing to the restricted diet it is perfectly satisfactory and normal to have an evacuation of the bowel only once every three to four days and that, provided plenty of fluids are taken, this never leads to any disturbance. Only in those patients who begin to fret after four days do we allow the use of a suppository. Patients who observe this rule find that after treatment they have a perfectly normal bowel action and this delights many of them almost as much as their loss of weight.

Investigating Dietary Errors

When the reason for a slight gain in weight is not immediately evident, it is necessary to investigate further. A patient who is unaware of having committed an error or is unwilling to admit a mistake protests indignantly when told he has done something he ought not to have done. In that atmosphere no fruitful investigation can be conducted; so we calmly explain that we are not accusing him of anything but that we know for certain from our not inconsiderable experience that something has gone wrong and that we must now sit down quietly together and try and find out what it was. Once the patient realizes that it is in his own interest that he play an active and not merely a passive role in this search, the reason for the set-hack is almost invariably discovered. Having been through hundreds of such sessions, we are nearly always able to distinguish the deliberate liar from the patient who is merely fooling himself or is really unaware of having erred.

Liars and Fools

When we see obese patients there are generally two of us present in order to speed up routine handling. Thus when we have to investigate a rise in weight, a glance is sufficient to make sure that we agree or disagree. If after a few questions we both feel reasonably sure that the patient is deliberately lying, we tell him that this is our opinion and warn him that unless he comes clean we may refuse further treatment. The way he reacts to this furnishes additional proof whether we are on the right track or not; we now very rarely make a mistake.

If the patient breaks down and confesses, we melt and are all forgiveness and treatment proceeds. Yet if such performances have to be repeated more than two or three times, we refuse further treatment. This happens in less than 1% of our cases. If the patient is stubborn and will not admit what he has been up to, we usually give him one more chance and continue it mean even though we have been unable to find the reason for his gain. In many such cases there is no repetition, and frequently the patient does then confess a few days later after he has thought things over.

The patient who is fooling himself is the one who has committed some trifling, offense against the rules but who has been able to convince himself that this is of no importance and cannot possibly account for the gain in weight. Women seem particularly prone to getting themselves entangled in such delusions. On the other hand, it does frequently happen that a patient will in the midst of a conversation unthinkingly spear an olive or forget that he has already eaten his breadstick.

A mother preparing food for the family may out of sheer habit forget that she must not taste the sauce to see whether it needs more salt. Sometimes a rich maiden aunt cannot be offended by refusing a cup of tea into which she has put two teaspoonful of sugar, thoughtfully remembering the patient's taste from previous occasions. Such incidents are legion and are usually confessed without hesitation, but some patients seem genuinely able to forget these lapses and remember them with a visible shock only after insistent questioning.

In these cases we go carefully over the day. Sometimes the patient has been invited to a meal or gone to a restaurant, naively believing that the food has actually been prepared exactly according to instructions. They will say: 'Yes, now that I come to think of it the steak did seem a bit bigger than the one I have at home, and it did taste better; maybe there was a little fat on it, though I specially told them to cut it all away". Sometimes the breadsticks were broken and a few fragments eaten, and "Maybe they were a little more than one". It is not uncommon for patients to place too much reliance on their memory of the diet-sheet and start eating carrots, beans or peas and then to seem genuinely surprised when their attention is called to the fact that these are forbidden, as they have not been listed.

Cosmetics

When no dietary error is elicited we turn to cosmetics. Most women find it hard to believe that fats, oils, creams and ointments applied to the skin are absorbed and interfere with weight reduction by HCG just as if they had been eaten. This almost incredible sensitivity to even such very minor increases in nutritional intake is a peculiar feature of the HCG method. For instance, we find that persons who habitually handle organic fats, such as workers in beauty parlors, masseurs, butchers, etc. never show what we consider a satisfactory loss of weight unless they can avoid fat coming into contact with their skin.

The point is so important that I will illustrate it with two cases. A lady who was cooperating perfectly suddenly increased half a pound. Careful questioning brought nothing to light. She had certainly made no dietary error nor had she used any kind of face cream, and she was already in the menopause. As we felt that we could trust her implicitly, we left the question suspended. Yet just as she was about to leave the consulting worn she suddenly stopped, turned and snapped her fingers. "I've got it" she said. This is what had happened : She had bought herself a new set of make-up pots and bottles and, using her fingers, had transferred her large assortment of cosmetics to the new containers in anticipation of the day she would be able to use them again after her treatment.

The other case concerns a man who impressed us as being very conscientious. He was about 20 lbs. overweight hut did not lose satisfactorily from the onset of treatment. Again and again we tried to find the reason but with no success, until one day he said: "I never told you this, but I have a glass eye. In fact, I have a whole set of them. I frequently change them, and every time I do that I put a special ointment in my eye socket. Do you think that could have anything to do with it?' As we thought just that, we asked him to stop using this ointment, and from that day on his weight-loss was regular.

We are particularly averse to those modern cosmetics which contain hormones, as any interference with endocrine regulations during treatment must be absolutely avoided. Many women whose skin has in the course of years become adjusted to the use of fat containing cosmetics find that their skin gets dry as soon as they stop using them. In such cases we permit the use of plain mineral oil, which has no nutritional value. On the other hand, mineral oil should not be used in preparing the food, first because of its undesirable laxative quality, and second because it absorbs some fat-soluble vitamins, which are then lost in the stool. We do permit the use of lipstick, powder and such lotions as are entirely free of fatty substances. We also allow brilliantine to be used on the hair but it must not be rubbed into the scalp. Obviously sun-tan oil is prohibited.

Many women are horrified when told that for the duration of treatment they cannot use face creams or have facial massages. They fear that this and the loss of weight will ruin their complexion. They can be fully reassured. Under treatment Normal fat is restored to the skin, which rapidly becomes fresh and turgid, making the expression much more youthful. This is a characteristic of the HCG method which is a constant source of wonder to patients who have experienced or seen in others the facial ravages produced by the usual methods of reducing. An obese woman of 70 obviously cannot expect to have her pied face reduced to normal without a wrinkle, but it is remarkable how youthful her face remains in spite of her age.

The Voice

Incidentally, another interesting feature of the HCG method is that it does not ruin a singing voice. The typically obese prima donna usually finds that when she tries to reduce her weight the timbre of her voice is liable to change, and understandably this terrifies her. Under HCG this does not happen; indeed, in many cases the voice improves and the breathing invariably does. We have had many cases of professional singers very carefully controlled by expert voice teachers, and they have been so enthusiastic that they now frequently send us patients.

Other Reasons for a gain

Apart from diet and cosmetics there can be a few other reasons for a small rise in weight. Some patients unwittingly take chewing gum, throat pastilles, vitamin pills, cough syrups etc., without realizing that the sugar or fats they contain may interfere with a regular loss of weight. Sex hormones or cortisone in its various modern forms must be avoided, though oral contraceptives are permitted. In fact the only self-medication we allow is aspirin for a headache, though headaches almost invariably disappear after a week of treatment, particularly if of the migraine type.

Occasionally we allow a sleeping tablet or a tranquilizer, but patients should be told that while under treatment they need and may get less sleep. For instance, here in Italy where it is customary to sleep during the siesta which lasts from one to four in the afternoon most patients find that though they lie down they are unable to sleep.

We encourage swimming and sun bathing during treatment, but it should be remembered that severe sunburn always produces a temporary rise in weight, evidently due to water retention. The same may be seen when a patient gets a common cold during treatment. Finally, the weight can temporarily increase - paradoxical though this may sound after an exceptional physical exertion of long duration leading to a feeling of exhaustion. A game of tennis, a vigorous swim, a run, a ride on horseback or a round of golf do not have this effect; but a long trek, a day of skiing, rowing or cycling or dancing into the small hours usually result in a gain of weight on the following day, unless the patient is in perfect training. In patients coming from abroad, where they always use their cars, we often see this effect after a strenuous day of shopping on foot, sightseeing and visits to galleries and museums. Though the extra muscular effort involved does consume some additional Calories, this appears to be offset by the retention of water which the tired circulation cannot at once eliminate them. I frequently change them, and every time I do that I put a special ointment in my eye socket. Do you think that could have anything to do with it?' As we thought just that, we asked him to stop using this ointment, and from that day on his weight-loss was regular.

Appetite-reducing Drugs

We hardly ever use amphetamines, the appetite-reducing drugs such as Dexedrin, Dexamil, Preludin, etc., as there seems to be no need for them during the HCG treatment. The only time we find them useful is when a patient is for impelling and unforeseen reason obliged to forego the injections for three to four days and yet wishes to continue the diet so that he need not interrupt the course.

Unforeseen Interruptions of Treatment

If an interruption of treatment lasting more than four days is necessary, the patient must increase his diet to at least 800 Calories by adding meat, eggs, cheese, milk to his diet after the third day, as otherwise he will find himself so hungry and weak that he is unable to go about his usual occupation. If the interval lasts less than two weeks the patient can directly resume injections and the 500-Calorie diet, but if the interruption lasts longer he must again eat normally until he has had his third injection.

When a patient knows beforehand that he will have to travel and he absent for more than four days, it is always better to stop injections three days before he is due to leave so that he can have the three days of strict dieting which are necessary after the last injection at home. This saves him from the almost impossible task of having to arrange the 500 Calorie diet while en route, and he can thus enjoy a much greater dietary freedom from the day of his departure. Interruptions occurring before 20 effective injections have been given are most undesirable, because with less than that number of injections some weight is liable to be regained. After the 20th injection an unavoidable interruption is merely a loss of time.

Muscular Fatigue

Towards the end of a full course when a good deal of fat has been rapidly lost, some patients complain that lifting a weight or climbing stairs requires a greater muscular effort than before. They feel neither breathlessness nor exhaustion but simply that their muscles have to work harder. This phenomenon, which disappears soon after the end of the treatment, is caused by the removal of Abnormal fat deposited between, in and around the muscles. The removal of this fat makes the muscles too long, and so in order to achieve a certain skeletal movement - say the bending of an arm - the muscles have to perform greater contraction than before. Within a short while the muscle adjusts itself perfectly to the new situation, but under HCG the loss of fat is so rapid that this adjustment cannot keep up with it. Patients often have to be reassured that this does not mean that they are "getting weak". This phenomenon does not occur in patients who regularly take vigorous exercise and continue to do so during treatment.

Massage

I never allow any kind of massage during treatment. It is entirely unnecessary and merely disturbs a very delicate process which is going on in the tissues. Few indeed are the masseurs and masseuses who can resist the temptation to knead and hammer Abnormal fat deposits. In the course of rapid reduction it is sometimes possible to pick up a fold of skin which has not yet had time to adjust itself, as it always does under HCG, to the changed figure. This fold contains its normal subcutaneous fat and may be almost an inch thick. It is one of the main objects of the HCG treatment to keep that fat there. Patients and their masseurs do not always understand this and hopefully give this fat a working over. I have seen such patients who were as black and blue as if they had received a sound thrashing.

In my opinion, massage, thumping rolling, kneading and shivering undertaken for the purpose of reducing Abnormal fat can do nothing but harm. We once had the honor of treating the proprietress of a high class institution that specialized in such antics. She had the audacity to confess that she was taking our treatment to convince her clients of the efficacy of her methods, which she had found useless in her own case. How anyone in his right mind is able to believe that fatty tissue can be shifted mechanically or be made to vanish by squeezing is beyond my comprehension. The only effect obtained is severe bruising. The torn tissue then forms scars, and these slowly contract making the fatty tissue even harder and more unyielding.

A lady once consulted us for her most ungainly legs. Large masses of fat bulged over the ankles of her tiny feet, and there were about 40 lbs. too much on her hips and thighs. We assured her that this overweight could be lost and that her ankles would markedly improve in the process. Her treatment progressed most satisfactorily but to our surprise there was no improvement in her ankles. We then discovered that she had for years been taking every kind of mechanical, electric and heat treatment for her legs and that she had made up her mind to resort to plastic surgery if we failed.

Re-examining the fat above her ankles, we found that it was unusually hard. We attributed this to the countless minor injuries inflicted by kneading. These injuries had healed but had left a tough network of connective scar-tissue in which the fat was imprisoned. Ready to try anything, she was put to bed for the remaining three weeks of her first course with her lower legs tightly strapped in unyielding bandages. Every day the pressure was increased. The combination of HCG, diet and strapping brought about a marked improvement in the shape of her ankles. At the end of her first course she returned to her home abroad. Three months later she came back for her second course. She had maintained both her weight and the improvement of her ankles. The same procedure was repeated, and after five weeks she left the hospital with a normal weight and legs that, if not exactly shapely, were at least unobtrusive. Where no such injuries of the tissues have been inflicted by inappropriate methods of treatment, these drastic measures are never necessary.

Blood Sugar

Towards the end of a course or when a patient has nearly reached his normal weight it occasionally happens that the blood sugar drops below normal, and we have even seen this in patients who had an abnormally high blood sugar before treatment. Such an attack of hypoglycemia is almost identical with the one seen in diabetics who have taken too much insulin, The attack comes on suddenly, there is the same feeling of light-headedness, weakness In the knees, trembling and unmotivated sweating; but under HCG hypoglycemia does not produce any feeling of hunger. All these symptoms are almost instantly relieved by taking two heaped teaspoonful of sugar.

In the course of treatment the possibility of such an attack is explained to those patients who are in a phase in which a drop in blood sugar may occur. They are instructed to keep sugar or glucose sweets handy, particularly when driving a car. They are also held to watch the effect of taking sugar very carefully and report the following day. This is important, because anxious patients to whom such an attack has been explained are apt to take sugar unnecessarily, in which case it inevitably produces a gain in weight and does not dramatically relieve the symptoms for which it was taken, proving that these were not due to hypoglycemia. Some patients mistake the effects of emotional stress for hypoglycemia. When the symptoms are quickly relieved by sugar this is proof that they were indeed due to an abnormal lowering of the blood sugar, and in that case there is no increase in the weight on the following day. We always suggest that sugar be taken if the patient is in doubt.

Once such an attack has been relieved with sugar we have never seen it recur on the immediately subsequent days, and only very rarely does a patient have two such attacks separated by several days during a course of treatment. In patients who have not eaten sufficiently during the first two days of treatment we sometimes give sugar when the minor symptoms usually felt during the first there days of treatment continue beyond that time, and in some cases this has seemed to speed up the euphoria ordinarily associated with the HCG method.

Fibroids

While uterine fibroids seem to be in no way affected by HCG in the doses we use, we have found that very large, externally palpable uterine myomas are apt to give trouble. We are convinced that this is entirely due to the rather sudden disappearance of fat from the pelvic bed upon which they rest and that it is the weight of the tumor pressing on the underlying tissues which accounts for the discomfort or pain which may arise during treatment. While we disregard even fair-sized or multiple myomas, we insist that very large ones be operated before treatment. We have had patients present themselves for reducing fat from their abdomen who showed no signs of obesity, but had a large abdominal tumor.

Gallstones

Small stones in the gall bladder may in patients who have recently had typical colics cause more frequent colics under treatment with HCG. This may be due to the almost complete absence of fat from the diet, which prevents she normal emptying of the gall bladder. Before undertaking treatment we explain to such patients that there is a risk of more frequent and possibly severe miles and that it may become necessary to operate. If they are prepared to take this risk and provided they agree to undergo an operation if we consider this imperative we proceed with treatment as after weight reduction with HCG the operative risk is consider ably reduced in an obese patient. In such cases we always give a drug which stimulates the flow of bile, and in the majority of cases nothing untoward happens. On the other hand, we have looked for and not found any evidence to suggest that the HCG treatment leads to the formation of gallstones as pregnancy sometimes does.

The Heart

Disorders of the heart are not as a rule contraindications. In fact, the removal of Abnormal fat - particularly from the heart- muscle and from the surrounding of the coronary arteries - can only be beneficial in cases of myocardial weakness, and many such patients are referred to us by cardiologists. Within the first week of treatment all patients - not only heart cases - remark that they have lost much of their breathlessness.

Coronary Occlusion

In obese patients who have recently survived a coronary occlusion we adopt the following procedure in collaboration with the cardiologist. We wait until no further electrocardiographic changes have occurred for a period of three months. Routine treatment is then started under careful control and it is usual to find a further electrocardiographic improvement of a condition which was previously stationary.

In the thousands of cases we have treated we have not once seen any sort of coronary incident occur during or shortly after treatment. The same applies to cerebral vascular accidents. Nor have we ever seen a case of thrombosis of any sort develop during treatment, even though a high blood pressure is rapidly lowered. In this respect, too, the HCG treatment resembles pregnancy.

Teeth and Vitamins

Patients whose teeth are in poor repair sometimes get more trouble under prolonged treatment, just as may occur in pregnancy. In such cases we do allow calcium and vitamin D, though not in an oily solution. The only other vitamin we permit is vitamin C, which we use in large doses combined with an antihistaminic at the onset of a common cold. There is no objection to the use of an antibiotic if this is required, for instance by the dentist. In cases of bronchial asthma and hay fever we have occasionally resorted to cortisone during treatment and find that triamcinolone is the least likely to interfere with the loss of weight, but many asthmatics improve with HCG alone.

Alcohol

Obese heavy drinkers, even those bordering on alcoholism, often do surprisingly well under HCG and it is exceptional for them to take a drink while under treatment. When they do, they find that a relatively small quantity of alcohol produces intoxication. Such patients say that they do not feel the need to drink. This may in part be due to the euphoria which the treatment produces and in part to the complete absence of the need for quick sustenance from which most obese patients suffer.

Though we have had a few cases that have continued abstinence long after treatment, others relapse as soon as they are back on a normal diet. We have a few "regular customers" who, having once been reduced to their normal weight, start to drink again though watching their weight. Then after some months they purposely overeat in order to gain sufficient weight for another course of HCG which temporarily gets them out of their drinking routine. We do not particularly welcome such cases, hut we see no reason for refusing their request.

Tuberculosis

It is interesting that obese patients suffering from inactive pulmonary tuberculosis can be safely treated. We have under very careful control treated patients as early as three months after they were pronounced inactive and have never seen a relapse occur during or shortly after treatment. In fact, we only have one case on our records in which active tuberculosis developed in a young man about one year after a treatment which had lasted three weeks. Earlier X-rays showed a calcified spot from a childhood infection which had not produced clinical symptoms. There was a family history of tuberculosis, and his illness started under adverse conditions which certainly had nothing to do with the treatment. Residual calcifications from an early infection are exceedingly common, and we never consider them a contraindication to treatment.

The Painful Heal

In obese patients who have been trying desperately to keep their weight down by severe dieting, a curious symptom sometimes occurs. They complain of an unbearable pain in their heels which they feel only while standing or walking. As soon as they take the weight off their heels the pain ceases. These cases are the bane of the rheumatologists and orthopedic surgeons who have treated them before they come to us. All the usual investigations are entirely negative, and there is not the slightest response to anti- rheumatic medication or physiotherapy. The pain may be so severe that the patients are obliged to give up their occupation, and they are not infrequently labeled as a case of hysteria. When their heels are carefully examined one finds that the sole is softer than normal and that the heel bone - the calcaneus - can be distinctly felt, which is not the case in a normal foot.

We interpret the condition as a lack of the hard fatty pad on which the calcaneus rests and which protects both the bone and the skin of the sole from pressure. This fat is like a springy cushion which carries the weight of the body. Standing on a heel in which this fat is missing or reduced must obviously be very painful. In their efforts to keep their weight down these patients have consumed this normal Structural fat.

Those patients who have a normal or subnormal weight while showing the typically obese fat deposits are made to eat to capacity, often much against their will, for one week. They gain weight rapidly but there is no improvement in the painful heels. They are then started on the routine HCG treatment. Overweight patients are treated immediately. In both cases the pain completely disappears in 10-20 days of dieting, usually around the 15th day of treatment, and so far no case has had a relapse, though we have been able to follow up such patients for years. We are particularly interested in these cases, as they furnish further proof of the contention that HCG + 500 Calories not only removes Abnormal fat but actually permits Normal fat to be replaced, in spite of the deficient food intake. It is certainly not so that the mere loss of weight reduces the pain, because it frequently disappears before the weight the patient had prior to the period of forced feeding is reached.

The Skeptical Patient

Any doctor who starts using the HCG method for the first time will have considerable difficulty, particularly if he himself is not fully convinced, in making patients believe that they will not feel hungry on 500 Calories and that their face will not collapse. New patients always anticipate the phenomena they know so well from previous treatments and diets and are incredulous when told that these will not occur. We overcome all this by letting new patients spend a little time in the waiting room with older hands, who can always be relied upon to allay these fears with evangelistic zeal, often demonstrating the finer points on their own body.

A waiting-room filled with obese patients who congregate daily is a sort of group therapy. They compare notes and pop back into the waiting room after the consultation to announce the score of the last 24 hours to an enthralled audience. They cross-check on their diets and sometimes confess sins which they try to hide from us, usually with the result that the patient in whom they have confided palpitatingly tattles the whole disgraceful story to us with a "But don't let her know I told you".

The Ratio of Pounds to Inches

An interesting feature of the HCG method is that, regardless of how fat a patient is, the greatest clrcumference -- abdomen or hips as the case may be is reduced at a constant rate which is extraordinarily close to 1 cm. per kilogram of weight lost. At the beginning of treatment the change in measurements is somewhat greater than this, but at the end of a course it is almost invariably found that the girth is as many centimeters less as the number of kilograms by which the weight has been reduced. I have never seen this clear cut relationship in patients that try to reduce by dieting only.

Preparing the Solution

Human chorionic gonadotrophin comes on the market as a highly soluble powder which is the pure substance extracted from the urine of pregnant women. Such preparations are carefully standardized, and any brand made by a reliable pharmaceutical company is probably as good as any other. The substance should be extracted from the urine and not from the placenta, and it must of course be of human and not of animal origin. The powder is sealed in ampoules or in rubber-capped bottles in varying amounts which are stated in International Units. In this form HCG is stable; however, only such preparations should he used that have the date of manufacture and the date of expiry clearly stated on the label or package. A suitable solvent is always supplied in a separate ampoule in the same package.

Once HCG is in solution it is far less stable. It may be kept at room-temperature for two to three days, but if the solution must be kept longer it should always be refrigerated. When treating only one or two cases simultaneously, vials containing a small number of units say 1000 I.U. should be used. The 10 cc. of solvent which is supplied by the manufacturer is injected into the rubber- capped bottle containing the HCG, and the powder must dissolve instantly. Of this solution 1 .25 cc. are withdrawn for each injection. One such bottle of 1000 I.U. therefore furnishes 8 injections. When more than one patient is being treated, they should not each have their own bottle but rather all be injected from the same vial and a fresh solution made when this is empty.

As we are usually treating a fair number of patients at the same time, we prefer to use vials containing 5000 units. With these the manufactures also supply 10 cc. of solvent. Of such a solution 0.25 cc. contain the 125 I.U. Which is the standard close for all cases and which should never be exceeded. This small amount is awkward to handle accurately (it requires an insulin syringe) and is wasteful, because there is a loss of solution in the nozzle of the syringe and in the needle. We therefore prefer a higher dilution, which we prepare in the following way: The solvent supplied is injected into the rubber capped bottle containing the 5000 I.U . As these bottles are too small to hold more solvent, we withdraw 5 cc., inject it into an empty rubber-capped bottle and add 5 cc. of normal saline to each bottle. This gives us 10 cc. of solution in each bottle, and of this solution 0.5 cc. contains 125 I. U. This amount is convenient to inject with an ordinary syringe.

Injecting

HCG produces little or no tissue-reaction, it is completely painless and in the many thousands of injections we have given we have never seen an inflammatory or suppurative reaction at the site of the injection.

One should avoid leaving a vacuum in the bottle after preparing the solution or after withdrawal of the amount required for the injections as otherwise alcohol used for sterilizing a frequently perforated rubber cap might be drawn into the solution. When sharp needles are used, it sometimes happens that a little bit of rubber is punched out of the rubber cap and can be seen as a small black speck floating in the solution. As these bits of rubber are heavier than the solution they rapidly settle out, and it is thus easy to avoid drawing them into the syringe.

We use very fine needles that are two inches long and inject deep intragluteally in the outer upper quadrant of the buttocks. The injection should if possible not be given into the superficial fat layers, which in very obese patients must be compressed so as to enable the needle to reach the muscle. Obviously needles and syringes must be carefully washed, sterilized and handled aseptically. It is also important that the daily injection should be given at intervals as close to 24 hours as possible. Any attempt to economize in time by giving larger doses at longer intervals is doomed to produce less satisfactory results.

There are hardly any contraindications to the HCG method. Treatment can be continued in the presence of abscesses, suppuration, large infected wounds and major fractures. Surgery and general anesthesia are no reason to stop and we have given treatment during a severe attack of malaria. Acne or boils are no contraindication the former usually clears up, and furunculosis comes to an end. Thrombophiebitis is no contraindication, and we have treated several obese patients with HCG and the 500 Calorie diet while suffering from this condition. Our impression has been that in obese patients the phlebitis does rather better and certainly no worse than under the usual treatment alone. This also applies to patients suffering from varicose ulcers which tend to heal rapidly.

Concluding a Course

When the three days of dieting after the last injection are over, the patients are told that they may now eat anything they please, except sugar and starch provided they faithfully observe one simple rule. This rule is that they must have their own portable bathroom-scale always at hand, particularly while traveling. They must without fail weight themselves every morning as they get out of bed, having first emptied their bladder. If they are in the habit of having breakfast in bed, they must weigh before breakfast.

It takes about 3 weeks before the weight reached at the end of the treatment becomes stable, i.e. does not show violent fluctuations after an occasional excess. During this period patients must realize that the so-called carbohydrates, that is sugar, rice, bread, potatoes, pastries etc, are by far the most dangerous. If no carbohydrates whatsoever are eaten, fats can be indulged in somewhat more liberally and even a small quantity of alcohol, such as a glass of wine with meals, does no harm, but as soon as fats and starch are combined things are very liable to get out of hand. This has to be observed very carefully during the first 3 weeks after the treatment is ended otherwise disappointments are almost sure to occur.

Skipping a Meal

As long as their weight stays within two pounds of the weight reached on the day of the last injection, patients should take no notice of any increase but the moment the scale goes beyond two pounds, even if this is only a few ounces, they must on that same day entirely skip breakfast and lunch but take plenty to drink. In the evening they must eat a huge steak with only an apple or a raw tomato. Of course this rule applies only to the morning weight. Ex-obese patients should never check their weight during the day, as there may be wide fluctuations and these are merely alarming and confusing.

It is of utmost importance that the meal is skipped on the same day as the scale registers an increase of more than two pounds and that missing the meals is not postponed until the following day. If a meal is skipped on the day in which a gain is registered in the morning this brings about an immediate drop of often over a pound. But if the skipping of the meal - and skipping means literally skipping not just having a light meal - is postponed the phenomenon clues not occur and several days of strict dieting may be necessary to correct the situation.

Most patients hardly ever need to skip a meal. If they have eaten a heavy lunch they feel no desire to eat their dinner, and in this case no increase takes place. If they keep their weight at the point reached at the end of the treatment, even a heavy dinner does not bring about an increase of two pounds on the next morning and does not therefore call for any special measures. Most patients are surprised bow small their appetite has become and yet how much they can eat without gaining weight. They no longer suffer from an abnormal appetite and feel satisfied with much less food than before. In fact, they are usually disappointed that they cannot manage their first normal meal, which they have been planning for weeks.

Losing more Weight

An ex-patient should never gain more than two pounds without immediately correcting this, but it is equally undesirable that more than two lbs. be lost after treatment, because a greater loss is always achieved at the expense of Normal fat.

Any Normal fat that is lost is invariably regained as soon as more food is taken, and it often happens that this rebound overshoots the upper two lbs. limit.

Trouble After Treatment

Two difficulties may be encountered in the immediate post treatment period when a patient has consumed all his Abnormal fat or when after a full course the injection has temporarily lost its efficacy owing to the body having gradually evolved a counter regulation, the patient at once begins to feel much more hungry and even weak. In spite of repeated warnings, some over-enthusiastic patients do not report this. However, in about two days the fact that they are being undernourished becomes visible in their faces, and treatment is then stopped at once. In such cases - and only in such cases - we allow a very slight increase in the diet, such as an extra apple, 150 grams of meat or two or three extra breadsticks during the three days of dieting after the last injection.

When Abnormal fat is no longer being put into circulation either because it has been consumed or because immunity has set in. This is always felt by the patient as sudden, intolerable and constant hunger. in this sense the HCG method is completely self-limiting. With HCG it is impossible to reduce a patient, however enthusiastic, beyond his normal weight. As soon as no more Abnormal fat is being issued the body starts consuming Normal fat, and this is always regained as soon as ordinary feeding is resumed. The patient then finds that the 23 lbs. he has lost during the last days of treatment are immediately regained. A meal is skipped and maybe a pound is lost. The next day this pound is regained, in spite of a careful watch over the food intake. In a few days a tearful patient is back in the consulting room, convinced that her case is a failure.

All that is happening is that the essential fat lost at the end 0f the treatment, owing to the patient's reluctance to report a much greater hunger, is being replaced. The weight at which such a patient must stabilize thus lies 2-3 lbs. higher than the weight reached at the end of the treatment. Once this higher basic level is established, further difficulties in controlling the weight at the new point of stabilization hardly arise.

Beware of Over-enthusiasm

The other trouble which is frequently encountered immediately after treatment is again due to over-enthusiasm. Some patients cannot believe that they can eat fairly normally without regaining weight.

They disregard the advice to eat anything they please except sugar and starch and want to play safe. They try more or less to continue the 500-Calorie diet on which they felt to well during treatment and make only minor variations, such as replacing the meat with an egg, cheese or a glass of milk. To their horror they find that in spite of this bravura their weight goes up. So, following instructions, they skip one meager lunch and at night eat only a little salad and drink a pot of unsweetened tea, becoming increasingly hungry and weak. The next morning they find that they have increased yet another pound. They feel terrible, and even the dreaded swelling of their ankles is back. Normally we check our patients one week after they have been eating freely, but these cases return in a few days. Either their eyes are filled with tears or they angrily imply that when we told them to eat normally we were just fooling them.

Protein Deficiency

Here too the explanation is quite simple. During treatment the patient has been only just above the verge of protein deficiency and has had the advantage of protein being fed back into his system I from the breakdown of fatty tissue. Once the treatment is over there is no more HCG in the body and this process no longer takes place. Unless an adequate amount of protein is eaten as soon as the treatment is over protein deficiency is bound to develop, and this inevitably causes the marked retention of water known as hunger- edema.

The treatment is very simple. The patient is told to eat two eggs for breakfast and a huge steak for lunch and dinner followed by a large helping of cheese and to phone through the weight the next morning. When these instructions are followed a stunned voice is heard to report that two lbs. have vanished overnight, that the ankles are normal but that sleep was disturbed, owing to an extraordinary need to pass large quantities of water. The patient having learned this lesson usually has no further trouble.

Relapses

As a general rule one can say that 60-70% our cases experience little or no difficulty in holding their weight permanently. Relapses may be due to negligence in the basic rule of daily weighing. Many patients think that this is unnecessary and that they can judge any increase from the fit of their clothes some do not carry their scale with them on a journey as it is cumbersome and takes a big bite out of their luggage-allowance when flying. This is a disastrous mistake, because after a course of HCG as much as 10 lbs. can be regained without any noticeable change in the fit of the clothes. The reason for this is that after treatment newly acquired fat is at first evenly distributed and does not show the former preference for certain parts of the body.

Pregnancy or the menopause may annul the effect of a previous treatment. Women who take treatment during one year after the last menstruation - that is at the onset of the menopause - do just as well as others, but among them the relapse rate is higher until the menopause is fully established the period of one year after the last menstruation applies only to women who are not being treated with ovarian hormones. If these are taken, the premenopausal period may be indefinitely prolonged.
Late teenage girls who suffer from attacks of compulsive eating have by far the worst record of all as far as relapses are concerned.

Patients who have once taken the treatment never seem to hesitate to come back for another short course as soon as they notice that their weight is once again getting out of hand. They come quite cheerfully and hopefully, assured that they can be helped again. Repeat courses are often even more satisfactory than the first treatment and have the advantage, as do second courses, that the patient already, knows that he will feel comfortable throughout.

Plan of a Normal Course

125 I.U. of HCG daily (except during menstruation) U.I. injections have been given.
Until 3rd injection forced feeding.

After 3rd injection 500 Calorie diet to be continued 72 hours after the last injection.

For the following 3 weeks all foods allowed except starch and sugar in any form (careful with very sweet fruit).

After 3 weeks very gradually add starch in small quantities, always controlled by morning weighing.

CONCLUSION

The HCG + diet method can bring relief to every case of obesity, but the method is not simple. It is very time consuming and requires perfect cooperation between physician and patient. Each case must be handled individually, and the physician must have time to answer questions, allay fears and remove misunderstandings. He must also check the patient daily. When something goes wrong he must at once investigate until he finds the reason for any gain that may have occurred. In most cases it is useless to hand the patient a diet-sheet and let the nurse give him a "shot."

The method involves a highly complex bodily mechanism, and even though our theory may be wrong the physician must make himself some sort of picture of what is actually happening; otherwise he will not be able to deal with such difficulties as may arise during treatment.

I must beg those trying the method for the first time to adhere very strictly to the technique and the interpretations here outlined and thus treat a few hundred cases before embarking on experiments of their own, and until then refrain from introducing innovations, however thrilling they may seem. In a new method innovations or departures from the original technique can only be usefully evaluated against a substantial background of experience with what is at the moment the orthodox procedure.

I have tried to cover all the problems that come to my mind. Yet a bewildering array of new questions keeps arising, and my interpretations are still fluid. In particular, I have never had an opportunity of conducting the laboratory investigations which are so necessary for a theoretical understanding of clinical observations, and I can only hope that those more fortunately placed will in time be able to fill this gap.

The problems of obesity are perhaps not so dramatic as the problems of cancer or polio, but they often cause life long suffering. How many promising careers have been ruined by excessive fat; how many lives have been shortened. If some way -however cumbersome - can be found to cope effectively with this universal problem of modern civilized man, our world will be a happier place for countless fellow men and women.

GLOSSARY

ACNE . . . Common skin disease in which pimples, often containing pus, appear on face, neck and shoulders.

ACTH . . . Abbreviation for adrenocorticotrophic hormone. One of the many hormones produced by the anterior lobe of the pituitary gland. ACTH controls the outer part, rind or cortex of the adrenal glands. When ACTH is injected it dramatically relieves arthritic pain, but it has many undesirable side effects, among which is a condition similar to severe obesity. ACTH is now usually replaced by cortisone.

ADRENALIN . . . Hormone produced by the inner part of the Adrenals. Among many other functions, adrenalin is concerned with blood pressure, emotional stress, fear and cold.

ADRENALS . . . Endocrine glands. Small bodies situated atop the kidneys and hence also known as suprarenal glands. The adrenals have an outer rind or cortex which produces vitally Important hormones, among which are Cortisone similar sub-stances. The adrenal cortex is controlled by ACTH. The inner part of the adrenals, the medulla, secretes adrenalin and is chiefly controlled by the autonomous nervous system.

ADRENOCORTEX... See adrenals.

AMPHETAMINES . . . Synthetic drugs which reduce the awareness of hunger arid stimulate mental activity, rendering sleep impossible. When used for the latter two purposes they are dangerously habit-forming. They do not diminish the body's need for food, but merely suppress the perception of that need. The original drug was known as benzedrine, from which modern variants such as dexedrine, dexamil, preludin, etc., have been derived. Amphetamines may help an obese patient to prevent a further increase in weight but are unsatisfactory for reducing, as they do not cure the underlying disorder and as their prolonged use may lead to malnutrition and addiction.

ARTERIOSCLEROSIS . . . Hardening of the arterial wall through the calcification of abnormal deposits of a fatlike substance known as cholesterol.

ASCHFIE1M-ZONDEK . . . Authors of a test by which early pregnancy can be diagnosed by injecting a woman's urine into female mice. The HCG present in pregnancy urine produces certain changes

236

in the vagina of these animals. Many similar tests, using other animals such as rabbits, frogs, etc. have been devised.

ASSIMILATE . . . Absorbed digested food from the intestines.

AUTONOMOUS . . . Here used to describe the independent or vegetative nervous system which manages the automatic regulations of the body.

BASAL METABOLISM . . . The body's chemical turnover at complete rest and when fasting. The basal metabolic rate is expressed as the amount of oxygen used up in a given time. The basal metabolic rate (BMR) is controlled by the thyroid gland.

CALORIE . . . The physicist's calorie is the amount of heat required to raise the temperature of 1 cc. of water by 1 degree Centigrade. The dieticiari's Calorie (always written with a capital C) is 1000 times greater. Thus when we speak of a 500 Calorie diet this means that the body is being supplied with as much fuel as would be required to raise the temperature of 500 liters of water by 1 degree Centigrade or 50 liters by 10 degrees. This is quite insufficient to cover the heat and energy requirements of an adult body. In the HCG method the deficit is made up from the Abnormal fat- deposits, of which 1 lb. furnishes the body with more than 2000 Calories. As this is roughly the amount lost every day, a patient under HCG is never short of fuel.

CEREBRAL . . . Of the brain. Cerebral vascular disease is a disorder concerning the blood - vessels of the brain, such as cerebral thrombosis or hemorrhage, known as apoplexy or stroke.

CHOLESTEROL . . . A fatlike substance contained in almost every cell of the body. In the blood it exists in two forms, known as free and esterified. The latter form is under certain conditions deposited in the inner lining of the arteries (see arteriosclerosis). No clear and definite relationship between fat intake and cholesterol-level in the blood has yet been established.

CHORIONIC . . . Of the chorion, which is part of the placenta or after-birth. The term chorionic is justly applied to HCG, as this hormone is exclusively produced in the placenta, from where it enters the human mother's blood and is later excreted in her urine.

COMPULSIVE EATING. . . A form of oral gratification with which a repressed sex-instinct is sometimes vicariously relieved. Compulsive eating must not be confused with the real hunger from which most obese patients suffer.

CONGENITAL . . . Any condition which exists at or before birth.

CORONARY ARTERIES . . . Two blood vessels which encircle the heart and supply all the blood required by the heart- muscle.

CORPUS LUTEUM . . . A yellow body which forms in the ovary at the follicle from which an egg has been detached. This body acts as an endocrine gland and plays an important role in menstruation and pregnancy. Its secretion is one of the sex hormones, and it is stimulated by another hormone known as LSH, which stands for luteum stimulating hormones. LSH is produced in the anterior lobe of the pituitary gland. LSI-I is truly gonadotrophic and must never he confused with HCG, which is a totally different substance, having no direct action on the corpus luteum.

CORTEX . . . Outer covering or rind. The term is applied to the outer part of the adrenals but is also used to describe the gray matter which covers the white matter of the brain.

CORTISONE . . . A synthetic substance which acts like an adrenal hormone. It is today used in the treatment of a large number of illnesses, and several chemical variants have been produced, among which are prednisone and triaincinolone.

CUSHING . . . A great American brain surgeon who described a condition of extreme obesity associated with symptoms of adrenal disorder. Cushing's Syndrome may be caused by organic disease of the pituitary or the adrenal glands but, as was later discovered, it also occurs as a result of excessive ACTH medication.

DIENCEPHALON . . . A primitive and hence very old part of the brain which lies between and under the two large hemispheres. In man the diencephalon (or hypothalamus) is subordinate to the higher brain or cortex, and yet it ultimately controls all that happens inside the body. It regulates all the endocrine glands, the autonomous nervous system, the turnover of fat and sugar. It seems also to be the seat of the primitive animal instincts and is the relay station at which emotions are translated into bodily reactions.

DIURETIC. . . . Any substance that increases the flow of urine.

DYSFUNCTION . . . Abnormal functioning of any organ, be this excessive, deficient or in any way altered.

EDEMA . . . An abnormal accumulation of water in the tissues.

ELECTROCARDIOGRAM . . . Tracing of electric phenomena taking place in the heart during each beat. The tracing provides information about the condition and working of the heart which is not otherwise obtainable.

ENDOCRINE . . . We distinguish endocrine and exocrine glands. The former produce hormones, chemical regulators, which they secrete directly into the blood circulation in the gland and from where they are carried all over the body. Examples of endocrine glands are the pituitary, the thyroid and the adrenals. Exocrine glands produce a visible secretion such as saliva, sweat, urine. There are also glands which are endocrine and exocrine. Examples are the testicles, the prostate and the pancreas, which produces the hormone insulin and digestive ferments which flow from the gland into the intestinal tract. Endocrine glands are closely inter dependent of each other, they are linked to the autonomous nervous system and the diencephalon presides over this whole incredibly complex regulatory system.

EMACIATED . . . Crossly undernourished.

EUPHORIA . . . A feeling of particular physical and mental well being.

FERAL . . . Wild, unrestrained.

FIBROID . . . Any benigi newgrowth of Connective tissue. When such a tumor originates from a muscle, it is known as a myoma. The most common seat of myomas is the uterus.

FOLLICLE . . . Any small bodily cyst or sac containing a liquid. Here the term applies to the ovarian cyst in which the egg is formed. The egg is expelled when a ripe follicle bursts and this is known as ovulation (see corpus luteurn).

FSH . . . Abbreviation for follicle-stimulating hormone. FSH is another (see corpus luteum) anterior pituitary hormone which acts directly on the ovarian follicle and is therefore correctly called a gonadotrophin.

GLANDS . . . See endocrine.

GONADOTROPHIN . . . See corpus luteum, follicle and FSH. Gonadotrophic literally means sex gland-directed. FSH, LSH and the equivalent hormones in the male, all produced in the anterior lobe of the pituitary gland, are true gonadotrophins. Unfortunately and confusingly, the term gonadotro phin has also been applied to the placental hormone of pregnancy known as human cborionic gonadotrophin (HCG). This hormone acts on the diencephalon and can only indirectly influence the sex-glands via the anterior lobe of the pituitary.

HCG . . . Abbreviation for human chorionic gonadotrophin

HORMONES . . . See endocrine.

HYPERTENSION . . . High blood pressure.

HYPOGLYCEMIA . . . A condition in which the blood sugar is below normal. It can he relieved by eating sugar.

HYPOPHYSIS . . . Another name for the pituitary gland.

HYPOTHESIS . . . A tentative explanation or speculation on how observed facts and isolated scientific data can be brought into an intellectually satisfying relationship of cause and effect. Hypotheses are useful for directing further research, but they are not necessarily an exposition of what is believed to be the truth. Before a hypothesis can advance to the dignity of a theory or a law, it must be confirmed by all future research. As soon as research turns up data which no longer fit the hypothesis, it is immediately abandoned for a better one.

LSH . . . See corpus luteum.

METABOLISM . . . See basal metabolism.

MIGRAINE . . . Severe half-sided headache often associated with vomiting.

MUCOID . . . Slime-like.

MYOCARDIUM . . . The heart-muscle.

MYOMA . . . See fibroid.

MYXEDEMA . . . Accumulation of a mucoid substance in the tissues which occurs in cases of severe primary thyroid deficiency.

NEOLITHIC . . . In the history of human culture we distinguish the Early Stone Age or Paleolithic, the Middlye Stone Age or Mesolithic and the New Stone Age or Neolithic period. The Neolithic period started about 8000 years ago when the first attempts at agriculture, pottery and animal domestication made at the end of the Mesolithic period suddenly began to develop rapidly along the road that led to modern civilization.

NORMAL SALINE . . . A low concentration of salt in water equal to the salinity of body fluids.

PHLEBITIS . . . An inflammation of the veins. When a blood- clot forms at the site of the inflammation, we speak of thrombophiebitis.

PITUITARY . . . A very complex endocrine gland which lies at the base of the skull, consisting chiefly of an anterior and a posterior lobe. The pituitary is controlled by the dienccphalon, which regulates the anterior lobe by means of hormones which reach it through small bloodvessels. The posterior lobe is controlled by nerves which run from the diencephalon into this part of the gland. The anterior lobe secretes many hormones, among which are those that regulate other glands such as the thyroid, the adrenals and the sex glands.

PLACENTA . . . The after-birth. In woman a large and highly complex organ through which the child in the womb receives its nourishment from the mother's body. It is the organ in which HCG is manufactured and then given off into the mother's blood.

PROTEIN . . . The living substance in plant and animal cells. Herbivorous animal can thrive on plant protein alone, but man must base some protein of animal origin (milk, eggs or flesh) to live healthily. When insufficient protein is eaten, the body retains water.

PSORIASIS . . . A skin disease which produces scaly patches. These tend to disappear during pregnancy and during the treatment of obesity by the HCG method.

RENAL . . . Of the kidney.

RESERPINE . . . An Indian drug extensively used in the treatment of high blood pressure and some forms of mental disorder.

RETENTION ENEMA . . . The slow infusion of a liquid into the rectum, from where it is absorbed and not evacuated.

SACRUM . . . A fusion of the lower vertebrate into the large bony mass to which the pelvis is attached.

SEDIMENTATION RATE . . . The speed at which a suspension of red blood cells settles out. A rapid settling out is called a high sedimentation rate and may be indicative of a large number of bodily disorders of pregnancy.

SEXUAL SELECTION . . . A sexual preference for individuals which show certain traits. If this preference or selection goes on generation after generation, more and more individuals showing the trait will appear among the general population. The natural environment has little or nothing to do with this process. Sexual selection therefore differs from natural selection, to which modern man is no longer subject because he changes his environment rather than let the environment change him.

STRIATION . . . Tearing of the lower layers of the skin owing to rapid stretching in obesity or during pregnancy. When first formed striae are dark reddish lines which later change into white scars.

SUPRARENAL GLANDS . . . See adrenals.

SYNDROME . . . A group of symptoms which in their association are characteristic of a particular disorder.

THROMBOPIILEBITIS . . . See phlebitis.

THROMBUS . . . A blood-clot in a blood-vessel.

TRIAMCINOLONE . . . A modern derivative of cortisone.

URIC ACID . . . A product of incomplete protein-breakdown or utilization in the body. When uric acid becomes deposited the gristle of the joints we speak of gout.

VARICOSE ULCERS . . . Chronic ulceration above the ankles due to varicose veins which interfere with the normal blood circulation in the affected areas.

VEGETATIVE . . . See autonomous.

VERTEBRATE . . . Any animal that has a back-bone.

Index

About the Author

Tobi Beck was born in Maryland, and has traveled the world most of her life. While serving in the Active Army as an Officer in the Military Police Corp. she spent more time deployed than at home. Her deployments included Somalia where she was the leader for well over two hundred combat missions. The extensive travel has taught her to see the world from multiple perspectives, and value the insight and variety that diversity offers. Her PhD is in Religious Philosophy and she holds a Juris Doctorate from Concord Law School. Currently she works for a high tech firm in the Midwest, serves her community as a foster parent and lives with her husband, dogs and cat.

www.ingramcontent.com/pod-product-compliance
Lightning Source LLC
Chambersburg PA
CBHW031504270326
41930CB00006B/239